中华传统经典养生术

（汉英对照）

(Chinese- English) Traditional and Classical Chinese Health Cultivation

Chief Producer	Li Jie	总策划	李 洁
Chief Compilers	Li Jie Xu Feng Xiao Bin Zhao Xiaoting	总主编	李 洁 许 峰 肖 斌 赵晓霆
Chief Translator	Han Chouping	总主译	韩丑萍
English Language Reviewer	Lawrence Lau	英译主审	劳伦斯·刘

逍

遥

功

Xiao Yao Gong (Free and Easy Exercise)

编著　肖　斌

Compiler　Xiao Bin

翻译　韩丑萍

Translator　Han Chouping

上海科学技术出版社

Shanghai Scientific & Technical Publishers

图书在版编目（CIP）数据

逍遥功：汉英对照 / 肖斌编著；韩丑萍译. —上
海：上海科学技术出版社，2015.5
（中华传统经典养生术）
ISBN 978-7-5478-2560-0

Ⅰ.①逍… Ⅱ.①肖… ②韩… Ⅲ.①气功–健身运
动–基本知识–汉、英 Ⅳ.①R214

中国版本图书馆CIP数据核字（2015）第042962号

逍遥功

编著 肖 斌

上海世纪出版股份有限公司
上 海 科 学 技 术 出 版 社 出版

中国图书进出口上海公司 发行

2015年5月第1版
ISBN 978-7-5478-2560-0/R·878

顾问委员会

Advisory Committee Members

主任

徐建光　陈凯先　严世芸　郑　锦

Directors

Xu Jianguang Chen Kaixian Yan Shiyun Zheng Jin

副主任

施建蓉　胡鸿毅　季　光　张怀琼　余小明　劳力行

Vice Directors

Shi Jianrong　Hu Hongyi　Ji Guang　Zhang Huaiqiong

Yu Xiaoming　Lao Lixing

学术顾问

严世芸　林中鹏　林　欣　李　鼎　俞尔科　王庆其

潘华信　潘华敏　姚玮莉　赵致平　李　磊

Academic Advisers

Yan Shiyun　　Lin Zhongpeng　　Shin Lin　　Li Ding　　Yu Erke

Wang Qingqi　Pan Huaxin　　Pan Huamin　Yao Weili

Zhao Zhiping　Li Lei

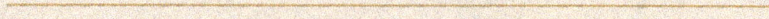

编纂委员会

Compilation Committee Members

总策划

李 洁

Chief Producer

Li Jie

总主编

李 洁 许 峰 肖 斌 赵晓霆

Chief Compilers

Li Jie   Xu Feng   Xiao Bin   Zhao Xiaoting

副总主编

孙 磊 陈昌乐 倪青根

Vice Chief Compilers

Sun Lei   Chen Changle   Ni Qinggen

总主译

韩丑萍

Chief Translator

Han Chouping

副主译

赵海磊

Vice Chief Translator

Zhao Hailei

项目资助

Acknowledgement

· 上海市新闻出版专项扶持资金项目

· 上海市中医药三年行动计划（2015—2018年）"基于〈中华气功史陈列馆〉科普教育基地为核心的〈中医气功文化平台〉建设"（项目编号：ZY3-WHJS-1-1010）

· Shanghai Press and Publication of special support funds program

· The Three-Year Action Plan for Chinese Medicine in Shanghai (2015–2018) on Construction of Qigong Cultural Platform in the Museum of Chinese Qigong History (Program No: ZY3-WHJS-1-1010)

序

　　欣闻上海市气功研究所编写的《中华传统经典养生术》丛书即将出版，这是中华原创医学文明传播的一件盛事，特致贺忱。

　　中华传统养生术源远流长，其中导引术更是重要的组成部分，它先于针、灸、药、医而形成，是中华民族最早用以防治疾病、养生保健的重要方法之一。现存早期文献《庄子》《吕氏春秋》《黄帝内经》以及考古发现《引书》《导引图》中均有关于养生导引及其具体方法的记载。此后绵绵数千年的历史长河中，中华养生导引术不断丰富、发展与创新，在自我实践中形成千门万法，在去伪存真中完善理论体系。20世纪后叶，古之导引术又以现代"气功"的面目再次席卷中华大地，并享誉海内外。时至今天，中华导引术仍然以其"人天合一"的整体观思想与丰富多姿的养生导引方法独立于世界自然医药之林，滋润着人类身心世界。事实表明，中华导引术已经形成为一门博大精深的学术体系。它所研究的是人之物质基础（精）与自组织能力（神）相互关系的规律，是关于"人"——这个地球上最复杂系统达到和谐与协调的一门学问。

　　我和上海市气功研究所相识逾30年，该所自20世纪70年代的中医研究所开始，气功与导引就是关注、研究的重点领域；80年代中期更名气功研究所后，更是全力着眼于现代气功的研究与中华导引术的弘扬。《中华传统经典养生术》是上海市气功研究所多年来所教授养生导引术、气功功法的汇编与总结，对于帮助学习、普及推广现代导引术具有较好的价值。希望此丛书的出版，能够进一步带动当前养生导引术在海内外的健康发展，推动中华优秀文化走向世界各地。

　　是以为序。

林中鹏

2015年3月

It is with great pleasure that I learn the *Traditional and Classical Chinese Health Cultivation* series compiled by the Shanghai Qigong Research Institute will be published soon. This means a lot to the spread of Chinese medical civilization.

Traditional Chinese health cultivation has a long-standing and well-established history. As an important part of health cultivation practice, Dao Yin exercise was used for disease prevention and treatment as well as life cultivation before acupuncture, moxibustion and herbal medicine. The recordings of *Dao Yin* and its specific exercise methods can be traced back to the *Zhuangzi, Lü Shi Chun Qiu* (The Annals of Lü Buwei), *Huang Di Nei Jing* (the Yellow Emperor's Inner Classic) and archaeologically unearthed books such as *Yin Shu* (a book on Dao Yin) and *Dao Yin Tu* (Dao Yin Diagram). After this, the thousands of years have witnessed the enrichment, progress and innovation of Chinese *Dao Yin* practice, coupled with emergence of numerous methods and perfection of its theoretical system. In late 20th century, the ancient *Dao Yin* exercise became exceptionally popular across China in the form of 'qigong'. Today, Chinese *Dao Yin* exercise remains flourish with its holistic 'Man-Nature Unity' idea and various exercise methods that benefit both body and mind. Facts show that there is a profound academic system behind Chinese *Dao Yin* exercise. This system studies the interactions between material foundation (essence) and self-organization ability (mind). In other words, it studies the way to achieve harmony and coordination of human being—the most complex system on earth.

I've established a friendship with the Shanghai Qigong Research Institute for 30 years. Ever since its founding in 1970s as a Research Institute of Chinese Medicine, qigong and *Dao Yin* have always been the research priorities of the Institute. The focuses on qigong and *Dao Yin* have been more highlighted in 1980s when the Institute was renamed as a Qigong Research Institute. I firmly believe that the

Traditional and Classical Chinese Health Cultivation series are of great significance in popularizing modern *Dao Yin* exercise. I sincerely wish the book series can further promote *Dao Yin* exercise at home and abroad and spread excellent Chinese culture.

For this, I wrote this forward.

Lin Zhongpeng
March 2015

前　言

气 以 臻 道

农历乙未早春，正是上海市气功研究所创建三十周年之际，恰逢气功学术发展枯木迎春之季。在此，我们谨向海内外气功学界发出倡言——构建现代气功"气以臻道"的学术思想。

所谓"气以臻道"，首先是指气功学术发展必须树立一个大方向，即中华传统文化精神的最高目标——"道"；其次是指通过对"气"的感性体验与理性认知，使生命更趋向"道"，与"道"合一。道者，规律、目标也；气者，方法、途径也；臻者，趋向、完善也。气-道共同构成"气以臻道"学术思想内核。其中气为实、主行，是具体之指；道为虚、主理，是抽象之喻。气因道而展，道由气而实；气以道归，道以气显；气借道而实际指归，道假气而理性论证。气功学术发展必须气、道并重，互印互证，理行一贯。两者既各尽其责、各擅其能，又有主从之别。"道"因标指形上本体而为万法归宗之源；"气"每描述形下万法而成法法生灭之流。"道"经思维抽象提炼，揭示规律、规则之理性思辨；"气"常直叙主观感觉，表述体会、觉受的感性认识。道-气，一主一从，一虚一实，构成中华气功学术思想的本质内涵。

"气以臻道"学术思想之主体是"道"，是指向真理之道路，是学术文化人文精神的体现，也是先人用身心去实践生命运化规律的心得体验，古人称为"内证之学"。"道"的外延旁及"功"和"术"，可以包括各种神秘现象、气功现象、特异现象，古人称为"神通法术"。当今，现代科学研究介入传统气功学术是时代进步的表现，它为我们观察生命奥秘打开了一个全新的视角。透过唯象的研究，重新激发起人类对生命的思考与敬重，重新挖掘出科技文明下的人文精神，而非单纯地将生命物质化，这才是现代科学介入传统气功的人

Xiao Yao Gong (Free and Easy Exercise) · 逍遥功

1

前言 · Preface

文价值所在。

　　有鉴于此，我们倡议构建现代气功研究之"气以臻道"学术思想，让中华传统文化与现代科学携起手来，揭示生命真谛，回归大道本源。

上海市气功研究所
2015年春

Advocacy for *Qi-Dao Harmony* in Modern Qigong Practice

　　The year 2015 is a Chinese new year of yin wood sheep (*Yi Wei* in Chinese). Wood, in Chinese culture on five elements (*Wu Xing*), is connected to the season of spring. The year 2015 also marks the 30th anniversary of the founding of Shanghai Qigong Research Institute. With a strong belief that the spring of 2015 will bring new hope to qigong study, we hereby advocate the concept of 'Qi-*Dao Harmony*' for its academic advance.

　　The term *Qi-Dao Harmony* has two underlying implications. First, it implies that *dao* is the ultimate goal of traditional Chinese culture and the general orientation for academic qigong advance. Second, it implies that our lives shall combine into one with the *dao* through perception and understanding of qi. In summary, this term means to achieve and perfect *dao* through qi exercise. The 'qi' here is weighted and refers to practice. The '*dao*' here is unweighted and refers to principles. Without *dao*, qi cannot extend; without qi, *dao* cannot become weighted. Qi finds its origin in *dao* and *dao* manifests itself in qi. Qi returns to *dao* eventually and *dao* supports qi theoretically. It's essential for people in academic qigong field to pay equal attention to qi and *dao*. The two have a principal-subordinate relationship. The metaphysical *dao* is the origin of all methods. The physical qi is the practice of all methods. *Dao* is about the abstract thinking and reveals the laws and rules. Qi is about the subjective feelings and tells experience and perception. Qi and *dao* constitute the essence of academic idea in Chinese qigong.

Let's get a deeper look into the concept of *Qi-Dao Harmony*. Also known as the 'learning of internal evidence', *dao* is the way to truth. It contains humanistic spirit and physical and mental experience of our ancestors. *Dao* extends to exercise (*gong*) and a variety of magic arts including mysterious, qigong and extrasensory phenomena. Today, modern scientific qigong research offers a new insight into the mysteries of life. The phenomenological research rekindles our reflection and respect towards life and enables us to re-discover humanism from modern civilization greatly impacted by science and technology. This is the real value of scientific research on traditional qigong in this materialized world.

To this end, we advocate the academic concept of '*Qi-Dao Harmony*' in modern qigong research. We believe the combination of traditional Chinese culture and modern science can help us to reveal the truth of life and return to the origin of the great *dao*.

Shanghai Qigong Research Institute
Spring 2015

编写说明

Words from the Compilers

中华传统养生术根植于中国传统哲学、中医学和养生学，是人体自我身心锻炼的有效方法。

随着倡导"主动健康"概念日益深入人心，具有调身、调息、调心功能的中华传统养生术，以其传统的养修理论、独特的身心效果蜚声海内外，引起世人的广泛关注。但近期国内外少见中国传统养生术的书籍出版，尤其没有成套、成系列的经典养生类作品问世，更缺乏英汉对照的专业著作。

上海中医药大学上海市气功研究所研究人员在前期研究工作基础上，精选中华传统经典养生术共八种，从历史源流、功法理论、特色要领、图解动作、分解说明与具体运用几方面进行中文编纂，由上海中医药大学中医英语专业人员进行翻译。并邀请专家进行中文审稿，邀请美国友三中医药大学Lawrence Lau先生审定英文翻译。

本套丛书详细地将八种中华经典养生术以图文并茂、视频摄像的形式记录下来，配以光盘，非常方便学习与传播，尤其便于海外养生爱好者以英语来学习。

本套丛书编纂过程中，得到上海市中医药三年行动计划（2015—2018年）"基于〈中华气功史陈列馆〉科普教育基地为核心的〈中医气功文化平台〉建设"（项目编号：ZY3-WHJS-1-1010）资助。

编者

Traditional Chinese health cultivation includes a variety of body-mind exercises, which are deeply rooted in ancient Chinese philosophy and medicine.

Today, the concept of 'health initiative (an ability to achieve physical, mental and social well-being)' has become well recognized.

Xiao Yao Gong (Free and Easy Exercise) · 逍 遥 功 · 编 写 说 明 · Words from the Compilers

2

Traditional Chinese health cultivation exercises are attracting worldwide attention because of their unique effects in regulating the breathing, body and mind. However, there are few books in this regard, especially the classical book series. There are even fewer bilingual Chinese-English versions of these books.

Based on their previous studies, research staff at the Shanghai Qigong Research Institute compiled eight traditional and classical health cultivation exercise methods, covering their history, theoretical foundation, characteristics and key principles, illustrated movements and application. Then these contents have been translated by professional interpreters at Shanghai University of Traditional Chinese Medicine. The Chinese version was reviewed by an expert team. The English version was reviewed by Dr. Lawrence Lau at the Yo San University of Traditional Chinese Medicine.

In addition to illustrations and videos are also available for readers, especially overseas health cultivation fans to learn.

This books series have been funded by the Three-Year Action Plan for Chinese Medicine in Shanghai (2015–2018) on Construction of Qigong Cultural Platform in the Museum of Chinese Qigong History (Program No: ZY3–WHJS–1–1010).

Compilers

目 录

Table of Contents

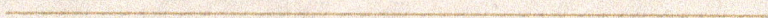

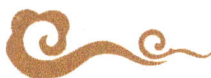

逍 遥 功 · *Xiao Yao Gong* (Free and Easy Exercise)

History

源流

逍遥功属道家导引功法，而道家以及后来归入道教的方士之术，可以说对养生气功的影响几乎是全方位的，几乎涵盖了所有的锻炼方法。如《庄子·刻意》云："吹呴呼吸，吐故纳新，熊经鸟申，为寿而已矣。此导引之士，养形之人，彭祖寿考者之所好也。"表明通过呼吸、吐纳、导引等的锻炼，可以达到健康长寿的目的。

Xiao Yao Gong falls under the category of Daoist *Dao Yin* exercise. It's known to all that Daoism and alchemy (closely connected to Daoism) greatly influenced health cultivation qigong in a multidirectional way. For example, the *Zhuang Zi Ke Yi* (Outer chapter 8, Zhuangzi) states, '...Breath in and out in various manners, exhale the old and inhale the new, walk like a bear and stretch their neck like a bird to achieve longevity. Such is the life favored by the scholars who practice *Dao Yin*, men who nourish the body and those who wish to live as long as Peng Zu[1]'. This indicates that breathing and *Dao Yin* exercise can benefit health and achieve longevity.

本功法称为逍遥功，其历史渊源可以追溯到先秦时期的庄子，逍遥之名取意自《庄子·逍遥游》，其云"藐姑射之山，有神人居焉。肌肤若冰雪，淖约若处子；不食五谷，吸风饮露；乘云气，御飞龙，而游乎四海之外；其神凝，使物不疵疠而年谷熟"。这正是道家功法性命双修，神游物外，逍遥自在，无为而治的写照。老庄道家思想的核心即是清净、自然、无为、柔和，都是自

---

1. Peng Zu: A legendary long-lived figure in China. He supposedly lived over 800 years in the Yin dynasty (1900 to 1066 BC). He was regarded as a saint in Taoism. The pursuit of eternity drugs by supporters of Taoism was highly influenced by Peng Zu. He is well known in Chinese culture as a symbol for long life.

然而然的体现在道家功法的演化之中，在气功中常用的松静自然，也出自道家思想。

Historically, *Xiao Yao Gong* can be traced far back to Zhuang Zi in late Warring States period (4th century BC). The name 'Xiao Yao' is from the *Zhuang Zi Xiao Yao You* (Inner chapter 1 of Zhuangzi, literally meaning free and easy wandering). This chapter states, 'He says that far way on Gu-she Mountain there dwells a spirit-like man with skin like icy snow, lovely and chaste as a young girl. He eats no grain, but sucks the wind and drinks the dew. He climbs up on the clouds and mist and wanders beyond the four seas riding a flying dragon. By concentrating his spirit, he protects creatures from sickness and plague and makes the harvest plentiful'. This description covers the essential Daoism beliefs — dual cultivation of inherent nature and life endowment, free oneself from the world, untroubled ease and govern by doing nothing that goes against the nature. The cores of Zhuangzi are pureness, at ease, inaction and softness. These ideas are often manifested in Daoist exercise, such as relaxation, tranquil and at ease in qigong practice.

本套功法是继承了道家养生导引的精华，结合传统医家导引，秉承道家逍遥游的精神而传播推广的养生导引功法，通过对本功法的习练，能进入一种松静至极的气功状态，不但能使人达到身逍遥（即身体松柔，动作灵活，气血通畅，脏腑调和），还能让人进入一种心逍遥（虚极静笃，神游物外）的美妙境界，最后达到祛病健身、身心和谐、益智延年的目标。它是由著名的气功医家董妙成老师继承和传授的，并经气功专家如马济人、林厚省、沈鹤年等进一步完善与发展，成为上海市气功研究所的传统经典功法之一。

Xiao Yao Gong has been developed on the basis of Daoist

Dao Yin, traditional health cultivation methods and spirit of *Xiao Yao You* (free and easy wandering). Practice of *Xiao Yao Gong* can help you to enter a relaxed tranquil qigong state, which not only involves a relaxed body (soft, flexible, smooth flow of qi and blood and harmony of zang-fu organs) but also a carefree mind (empty yourself of everything, let the mind become still and you free yourself from the world). Over time, you can achieve wellness and longevity. Inherited by Qigong master Dong Miao-cheng and further developed by qigong experts Ma Ji-ren, Lin Hou-sheng and Shen He-nian, *Xiao Yao Gong* has become one of the classical exercises in Shanghai Qigong Research Institute.

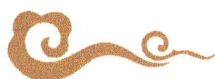

逍　遥　功　　•　　*Xiao Yao Gong* (Free and Easy Exercise)

理
论
基
础

性 命 双 修

Dual cultivation of inherent nature and life endowment (*Xing Ming Shuang Xiu*)

性指人的心性、思想、秉性、性格、精神等。命指人的身体、生命、能量、命运、物质等。性命双修也就是指"神形兼修"、心身全面修炼。《中和集》《性命圭旨》等内丹典籍都有关于"性命双修"的论述。《性命圭旨》说:"何谓之性? 元始真如,一灵炯炯是也。何为之命? 先天至精,一气氤氲是也。"又说:"性之造化系乎心,命之造化系乎身。"陈撄宁大师说:"性即是吾人之灵觉,命即是吾人之生机。"可谓既深刻,又生动。人的生命实际上是两个生命即精神生命和生理生命的双重融合,人们通常说健康就是要身心健康,亏其一即残缺不全。所以性命二字高度概括了人生的两大要素。

The first word *Xing* covers one's mind, thought, disposition, temperament and spirit. The second word *Ming* covers one's body, life, energy, fate and material things. Dual cultivation of inherent nature and life endowment can also be understood as body-mind cultivation. This idea was discussed in classics on internal alchemy such as the *Zhong He Ji* (Essays on Harmony) and *Xing Ming Gui Zhi* (Principles of Inherent Nature and Life Endowment). The *Xing Ming Gui Zhi* states, 'What is *Xing*? It's the innate disposition. What is Ming? It's the congenital essence or life endowment'. The text also states, 'the making of innate disposition is associated with the mind, and the making of life endowment with the body'. Chen Yingning (1880–1969), an influential Taoist figure in last century, once explained the two words in a vivid but profound way, '*Xing* is our spirituality and *Ming* is our vitality'. Our life covers physical and mental aspects. Health is a state of complete physical and mental well-being. Consequently, the two words (*Xing Ming*) summarized the two major elements of human life.

道教吸收了儒佛两家的心性学说,又发扬了自家传统的性命学说,遂形成性命双修的修炼理论。由此,我们可以将性命双修分为性功与命功两种,性功是道教与儒、佛相通的地方,而命功则是道教独有的传统,不讲命功,不是道教。陈撄宁大师认为,仙道贵生、乐生、重生、追求长生,所以它是生本主义,这正是道家最具特色的地方。他认为性命相依,命为重。他用灯作比喻,灯油是命,灯光是性;有灯无油,灯必不能发光;徒有灯油而不能发光,则不能显现油灯照明之用;修道之意在教人积足油量,并教以点灯之法,则人生必充满光辉。

Daoist exercise integrates the *Xin* (heart) *Xing* (inherent nature) doctrine in Buddhism and Confucianism into its *Xing* (inherent nature) *Ming* (life endowment) theory. As a result, the dual cultivation here contains exercise for inherent nature and exercise for life endowment. The former shares common features with Buddhism and Confucianism, the latter is unique to Daoism. Chen Ying-ning believed that one needs to cherish his life, live the best possible life and seek ways to achieve health and longevity. Personally he valued *Ming* more than *Xing*. Taking a lamp for example, he described *Ming* as the lamp oil and *Xing* as the lamp light. A lamp cannot give out light without oil; lamp oil cannot produce light without the lamp. Only with abundant lamp oil and correct way to ignite the lamp, can we have a bright life.

不同养生流派对"性""命"的理解及对两者的关系的认识不尽相同,但大多数认为性命一体,神形相依,主张"性命双修",即精神与形体同时修炼,只有形与神俱,才能延年益寿。性命一词,原指"人性"和"天命",是性与命的统一。后来,人们赋予它新的内涵,即指修性与养命、"性功"与"命功"的有机结合。在修养顺序上,有的主张"先性后命",也有主张"先命后性"。其修养原则为"性为主导,命为基础",以静为主,以动为辅,性命合一。其方法,以静养神,以动养形,即以静坐、行气、存神、诵经养神;以导引、按摩、散步、登涉养形。其根本宗旨,是以调动人体精、气、神的运化、聚合,达到形神永固、身心两健。性命双修成为人们养生保健、延年益寿的指导思想和方法论原则。

Although different health cultivation schools have different understandings regarding *Xing* and *Ming* and their interactions, they all agreed that health and longevity needs dual cultivation of inherent nature and life endowment. Originally, the word *Xing Ming* means human nature and fate. Later, it refers to cultivation of inherent nature and nurturing life. As for the cultivation sequence, some proposed '*Xing* first, *Ming* second' and some proposed '*Ming* first, *Xing* second'. The cultivation principle is to use *Xing* as the leader and use *Ming* as the foundation, i.e., more inner cultivation than body movements. More specifically, this exercise aims to nurture the mind by seated meditation (*Jing Zuo*), circulating qi, preserving spirit and chanting; to nurture the body by *Dao Yin*, massage, walking and mountain climbing. The fundamental purpose is to activate and exercise our essence, qi and spirit to obtain body-mind wellness.

心理健康与生理健康同时并重。不但要追求强健体魄,也要追求健全的心理素质,使精神生命和生理生命两个方面都得到活泼的发展,这才能有真正的幸福人生。《性命圭旨》中说"神不离气,气不离神""性不离命,命不离性"。以生理变化心理，以心理变化生理。体弱多病者先从命功入手，炼精化气，祛病健身，然后心神安定，炼气化神，炼神还虚，提高精神境界。心理脆弱或心性不定者，则先从性功入手，炼己筑基，排除私心杂念，调整心理平衡，提高追求层次，开拓心胸情怀，然后配合炼气，方能得到良好的效用。性功与命功可以在不同时候有不同侧重，但要互相带动，共同长进。

Mental health is equally important to physical health. It's important to have a sound mind in a sound body, because true happiness lies in mental and physical health. The *Xing Ming Gui Zhi* mentions, 'mind and qi are inseparable and so are *Xing* and *Ming*'. We can use the body to transform our mind or vice versa. Those with a weak constitution should start with active physical exercise to transform essence into qi, and then follow this with inner cultivation to transform qi into spirit. Those with psychological fragility or concentration difficulty should start with inner cultivation to cleanse the mind, remove distracting thoughts and elevate spiritual levels, and then follow this with and physical exercise. Active physical exercises and inner cultivation can be stressed in different periods of time; however, they are mutually promoted.

性命双修要循序渐进，由低到高，由浅入深。内丹家有"初关、中关、上关"之说，有"先摄心修性，次炼化精气修命，最后粉碎虚空"之说，其要不出初级、中级、高级三大阶段，次弟而上，不可躐等（逾越）。无论心灵的净化、境界的提升，还是气血的调适、体质的强化，都不是一蹴而就的事，要勤学苦练，长期坚持，不断体悟和反省，才能渐入佳境。当然渐中有顿，这是自然得来，不可强求。

Dual cultivation of inherent nature and life endowment needs a step-by-step plan. According to internal alchemy, there are three stages — primary, intermediate and advanced. Some scholars believe you need to cultivate your inherent nature first, then conduct active physical exercise to accumulate essence and qi and finally enter the utmost emptiness. It's unlikely to cleanse the mind, elevate the spiritual realm and harmonize qi and blood overnight. Only by regular exercise, strenuous effort and continuous self-reflection, can you naturally accomplish the above goals.

内 炼 精 气 神

Internal exercise of essence (*Jing*), qi and spirit (*Shen*)

养生，主要养的就是人的"精、气、神"。古代养生家遵循正确的修炼方法，往往能够获得健康和高寿。《灵枢·本藏》云："人之血气精神者，所以奉生而周于性命者也。"（人体血气精神的相互为用，是奉养形体，维护生命的根本）可见古人对这三方面的调护、摄养极为重视。

Nurturing life (*Yang Sheng*) or health cultivation simply means to nurture essence, qi and spirit. Ancient scholars who practice health cultivation could obtain health and longevity through correct exercise methods. The *Ling Su Ben Zang* (Chapter 47 of the Spiritual Pivot) states, 'Blood, qi and spirit are essential to nurture our life and maintain vital activities'.

那什么是精、气、神？精、气、神本是古代哲学中的概念，是指形成宇宙万物的原始物质，含有元素的意思。中医认为精、气、神是人体生命活动的根本。在古代讲究养生的人，都把

"精、气、神" 称为人身的三宝，如人们常说："天有三宝日、月、星；地有三宝水、火、风；人有三宝神、气、精。" 所以保养精、气、神是健身养生、延缓衰老的主要原则，尤其是当精、气、神逐渐衰退变化，人已步入老年的时候就更应该珍惜此 "三宝"，古人对这点是非常重视的。

What are essence, qi and spirit? Originally they are philosophical concepts, referring to primordial matter or elements that formed all things in the universe. In Chinese medicine, essence, qi and spirit are the material foundation for vital activities. Ancient people who practice health cultivation consider essence, qi and spirit as three treasures of the body. As the saying goes, 'the three treasures of the heaven are Sun, Moon and Stars; the three treasures of the earth are water, fire and wind; and three treasures of man are spirit, qi and essence'. Evidently the main principle to stay healthy, nurture life and delay aging is to preserve essence, qi and spirit, especially for the elderly with gradual decline in these three treasures.

所谓 "精"，就是指人体一切精微物质，有先后天之分。先天之精就是指元精，包括生殖之精（包含遗传信息的物质）。元精是人体生长发育的基础物质，它来自父母的精血，是构成人体生命活动的原始精微物质，元精随着人体生长发育，逐渐产生生殖之精。后天之精主要包括五脏六腑内所贮藏的精华物质，血液、津液和各种内分泌液等。气功锻炼能使先天和后天之精逐渐充养，就能提高人体精力和生殖能力。

Essence is nutrient substance of life. Congenital essence refers to primordial essence and inherited from one's parents (including genetic information), i.e., material foundation for human growth and development. Acquired essence refers to essential nutrients stored in five-zang and six-fu organs, including blood, body fluids and all kinds of secretion. Qigong practice can supplement both congenital and acquired essence and thus improve vigor and reproductive capacity.

所谓"气"就是指人体的生命活力，也有先天后天之分。先天之气就是指元气，又叫原气、真气，古代常称"炁"。所谓元气可理解为人体的生命力、免疫力、康复力，就是人体生命活动的动力。后天之气主要包括五脏六腑的功能活动，经络系统的功能活动和具有温养功能的卫气，以及具有营养成分的营气等。因此，气功锻炼能使先后天之气逐渐充足，就能增强人体的免疫功能和生理功能。对提高体力、增强体质、养生保健、延衰防老尤为重要。

Qi is the vital force of life. Congenital qi, also known as *Yuan*-primordial qi or *Zhen*-genuine qi, can be understood as human vitality, immunity or recuperative ability. Acquired qi includes functional activities of zang-fu organs and meridians, *wei*-defense qi that warms and defends the body and ying-nutrients qi that nurtures the body. Qigong exercise can gradually supplement acquired qi, boost the physiological functions and immune system and thus increase body constitution, promote health and delay aging.

所谓"神"就是人体意识、思维和智慧，与心和脑的关系最为密切。中医认为"心藏神""脑为元神之府"。神有先后天之分，先天之神就是指元神，可以理解为一种最原始的灵性。后天之神就是指识神，指通过各种学习以后所获得的知识、觉知和思辨力。所以，养生气功锻炼能使先后天之神逐渐旺盛，就能养成良好的心态，调节心理功能，提高大脑功能，对开发智力、发挥潜能、改善睡眠、增强记忆、预防痴呆等有较好作用。

Shen-spirit refers to mental consciousness, thought and wisdom. It is most closely associated with the heart and brain. In Chinese medicine, the heart stores spirit and brain houses spirit. Congenital *Shen* refers to primordial spirituality. Acquired *Shen* refers to knowledge perception and critical thinking ability through learning. Qigong exercise can supplement acquired *Shen*, cultivate a good mental state, regulate emotions, develop intelligence, increase memory and prevent dementia.

中国养生学乃至中国哲学,往往是神物一元的,并不存在意识和物质的对立。"神物"之间,由"气"来统一为一体。精、气、神构成中国传统养生和生命学说的重要部分。《太平经》说:"神者受之于天,精者受之于地,气者受之于中和。"三者统一于气,并互相增强和促进。通过行气导引的方法,如一般人可以通过合理运动、气功练习,道家通过内丹修炼,佛家通过静坐禅定等方法,来增强元气,进一步促进化生精、神,达到精、气、神的统一和圆满,成就养生的最高境界。

From the perspective of Chinese philosophy and health cultivation, spirit and essence attribute oneness. In other words, spirit and essence are united by qi. These three treasures play a key role in life theory and traditional Chinese health cultivation. The *Tai Ping Jing* (The Scripture on Great Peace) states, 'spirit is endowed by the heaven, essence by the earth and qi by harmony'. For ordinary people, yuan-primordial qi can be supplemented by appropriate exercise and qigong practice. For Daoist priests, yuan-primordial qi can be supplemented by internal alchemy. For Buddhist monks, yuan-primordial qi can be supplemented by meditation. All these methods can promote, transform and generate essence, qi and spirit and accomplish the highest state of health cultivation.

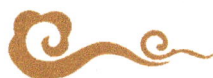

逍 遥 功　·　*Xiao Yao Gong* (Free and Easy Exercise)

Characteristics and Essential Principles

特色与要领

功 法 特 色

Characteristics of *Xiao Yao Gong*

本功法是在继承了古代道家养生导引术的基础上，结合了传统医学脏腑导引的精华，秉承了道家逍遥自在，遨游天地的心法意境而成的传统导引类功法，具有以下特色。

Based on the spirit of free and easy wandering and ancient Daoist *Dao Yin* exercise, *Xiao Yao Gong* also absorbs the quintessence of traditional Zang-fu *Dao Yin* exercise. Its characteristics are summarized as follows:

松
Relaxation (*Song*)

松之一字始终贯穿与整套功法之中，在练功中不但要做到形松、体松，还要求做到心松、意松，要在身心两方面避免紧张，消除紧张，使全身处于放松舒适的状态之中。

Relaxation runs through the exercise of *Xiao Yao Gong*. It's essential to relax both the body and mind during qigong practice.

静
Tranquil (*Jing*)

本功法在练习时强调静心凝神，集中注意力，克服心中纷起的杂念, 使身心处于一种安定祥和的状态, 所谓心定则气和, 气和则血顺, 血顺则精足而神旺, 精足神旺者, 内气充盈, 疾病自然消除。

A tranquil state is important for the exercise of *Xiao Yao Gong*. This means you need to concentrate your mind and get rid of distracting thoughts. We know that a tranquilized mind harmonizes qi, which in turn circulates blood. Smooth flow of blood provides the material foundation for our mental activities. Abundant internal qi can help us to remove diseases.

圆
Roundness (*Yuan*)

本功法的动作处处体现了一个 "圆" 字, 外形上没有走直线或有棱角的地方, 所谓无处不圆, 在形体动作上要求圆通灵活, 在心意上要求圆明周遍。

The body movements of *Xiao Yao Gong* are full of roundness. There are no straight lines or rough edges in physical appearance. What's more, roundness is not only in body movements but also in mental intention.

柔
Softness (*Rou*)

本功法动作柔和优美, 身体和骨节没有僵硬之处, 但又处处体现出内在的韧性, 并无软弱散漫之弊。

The body movements of *Xiao Yao Gong* are gentle, elegant but tenacious. There's no stiffness or rigidity in the joints and body.

缓
Slowness (*Huan*)

本功法动作缓慢，心态祥和宁静，让呼吸、意识与动作相结合，使三调相互融合，慢慢进入一种逍遥自在的练功境界。

Xiao Yao Gong involves unhurried body movements and a peaceful serene mind. Integration of breathing, mental consciousness and body movements can gradually take you to a free and easy qigong state.

功 法 要 领
Essential principles of *Xiao Yao Gong*

松静自然，舒缓圆活
Relaxation, Tranquil, Ease and Roundness

松静自然，即体松心静，这是气功锻炼的基本原则。是指在气功锻炼的具体操作过程中，都必须强调在以身体放松和心理放松的条件下进行。松，首先是某些紧张状态得到解除，练功中所以用这个字，是意味着练功过程中，使自己有意识地处于一种不紧张的、舒服轻松状态。而静是指心神的宁静祥和，注意力集中，心中没有各种杂念纷起，如神仙般逍遥自在。

It's essential to have a relaxed body and tranquil mind in qigong practice. In other words, qigong practice requires relaxation of both the body and mind. Relaxation begins with relief of stress. Tranquil refers to serenity, carefree and mental concentration without distracting thoughts.

本功法要求动作舒展柔和，速度缓慢均匀，姿态圆活灵动。配合呼吸的舒畅细匀，意识的宁静祥和，以期达到调和气血，调理脏腑的作用。

Ease and roundness are more for the body movements. Natural breathing, a tranquil mind and even, unhurried and flexible movements can harmonize qi and blood and benefit the zang-fu organs.

动静结合，炼养相兼
Combining body movements with inner cultivation and exercise with nourishment

动与静是对立的统一，能够相互影响，相互促进，相互转化，两者结合有利于气功修炼。本功法属导引功，在练动功时，要求动中有静，外形运动而神意安静，意念集中，此即所谓动中寓静。故动与静的有机结合，既有益于外在的形体运动，又有益于内气的聚集与运行，能够有效地提高练功效果。

Body movements and inner cultivation are unity of opposites. They interact and transform into each other. The two are both needed in qigong practice. As a *Dao Yin* exercise, *Xiao Yao Gong* requires tranquil inner cultivation during active physical exercise. Integration of the two can benefit the body movements and allows gathering and circulation of internal qi and thus improve the exercise result.

练养相兼，是指练功与调养并重，即练中有养，又练又养，这对于体质较差及慢性病患者尤其重要。练，是指练功过程，即合理的选择功法、练功强度和练功周期，认真踏实地修炼。养，主要是指练功必须与休整、调护身心，休养生息相结合，做到张弛有度，而不应无休止地练。

Combined exercise and nourishment is especially important for those with a weak constitution or having chronic conditions. Exercise means to practice regularly with certain intensity. Nourishment means to recuperate, nourish essence, qi and spirit during exercise or in daily living. Good exercise results come from a balanced exercise and nourishment.

意气相依，循序渐进
Mind (*Yi*)-qi interdependence and practice step by step

"意"是指练功中意念的运用，"气"这里是指呼吸之气和练功中内气运行的感觉。意与气，此两者在关系上，不能强调以意为主或以气为主，而是要互相依存，相互依恋。当呼吸逐渐变得深长细匀，是在练功过程中情绪安宁，意念集中的基础上慢慢出现的。所谓"心平气和""息调则心定，心定则息调"，心意识慢慢与呼吸之气相融相合，并进而引发内气的感触，这就是意气相依。

The *mind* here means the mental intention. The *qi* here refers to breathing and sensation of internal qi flowing. Mind and qi are interdependent. Deep and even breathing comes from a tranquil concentrated mind. This is what we call 'mind-qi harmony' and 'an even breathing leads to a tranquil mind and vice versa'. Mind-qi interdependence means internal qi is activated by integrated breathing and mental intention.

循序渐进是指在气功锻炼过程中，要根据功法的要求，认真地去做，并且根据自己身体的实际情况，具体地去领会各种锻炼方法的不同作用，分别在什么情况下应用怎样的方法，不断总结经验，从调身入手，结合调息，再结合调心，步步深入，层层递进，以达到进入忘形无我的气功状态。

It's important to practice qigong step by step — start by regulating the body, then breathing and finally the mind. Associated factors include individual constitution and requirements and functions of the exercise. Since overexertion may do harm to the body, it's advisable to exercise in moderation.

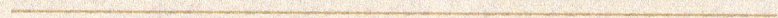

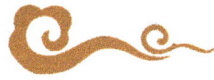

逍 遥 功　　•　　*Xiao Yao Gong* (Free and Easy Exercise)

Movements of *Xiao Yao Gong*

功法操作

基 础 操 作

Basic Movements

基本姿势
Basic posture

［要求］上身直而松，双膝不超过脚尖。

[Tips] Let you upper body relaxed and straightened and do not let your knees go past your toes.

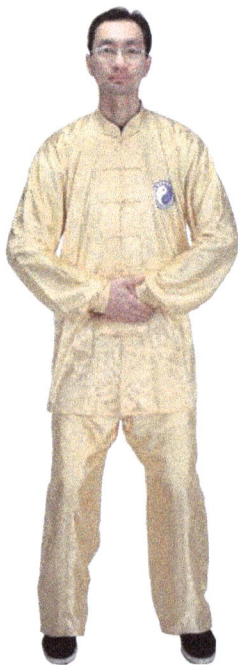

两脚平行站立与肩等宽，两手相叠抱丹田，双膝微屈下坐，成高位站桩。

Stand with your feet about shoulder-width apart, place the overlapped hands over Dantian and slightly flex the knee to make a high-position *Zhan Zhuang*.

基本姿势图　Basic posture

预备势
Preparation posture

两脚并拢，松静站立，凝神息虑，虚领顶劲，含胸拔背，两臂松垂于身体两侧，心里默念 "松" – "静"、"松" – "静"……

Put your feet together, stand in relaxation and tranquil, empty and concentrate your mind, pull up your Baihui (DU 20)[1] point on the top of your head, tuck in the chest, pull up the back, drop arms on both sides of the body and silently read *Song* (Relax) — *Jing* (Tranquil).

起势
Starting posture

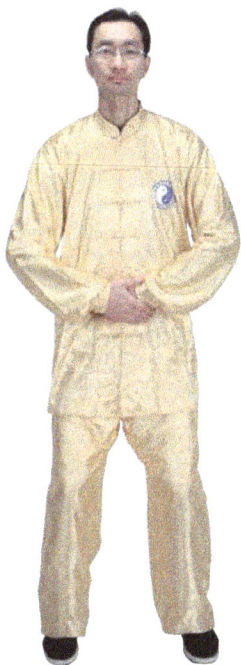

身体缓缓下沉，屈膝半坐，左脚向左平开一步，与肩等宽，身体慢慢站直。两掌外旋，缓缓向前合拢，划两个半圆，两手掌相叠置于肚脐之上，右手盖左手，同时屈膝下坐成高位站桩，静养1分钟。

Slightly sink the body, flex the knees (to make a half-sitting position), move the left feet one step to the left to shoulder-width part and slowly stand up straight. Turn the palms outward, slowly extend the palms forward, and fold the palms to draw two half circles. Place the overlapped palms (the right hand on top of the left hand) over the umbilicus and flex the knee to make a high-position *Zhan Zhuang*. Keep the posture for one minute.

起势图　Starting posture

---

1. At the junction of a line connecting the apices of the ears (in the middle).

具 体 操 作
Individual Movements

第一势　吐纳炼丹
Movement # 1　Strengthen *Dantian* through breathing

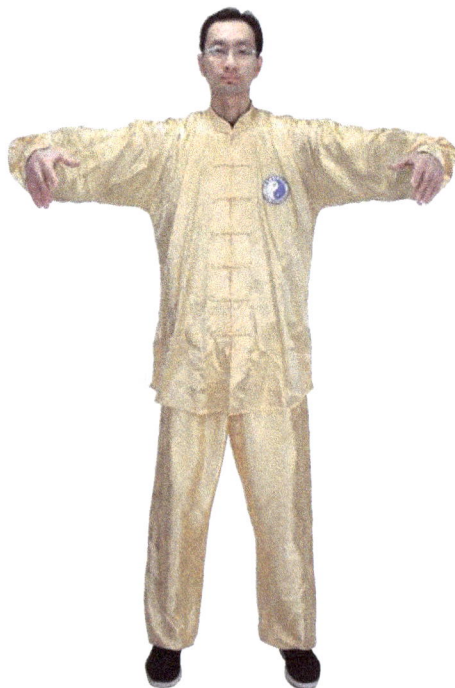

图 1-1　Fig 1-1

　　吸气，两臂从丹田部位向两侧45°缓缓提起，掌心向下，至手掌与肩平，两臂微曲，如抱一个缓缓涨大的气球。

　　Inhalation: Slowly lift the arms (palms downward) from Dantian to both sides (at an angle of 45°) until the palms are at the level of the shoulders. Slightly flex the arms as if holding a gradually inflated balloon.

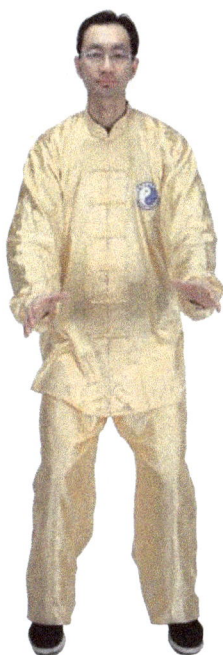

呼气，两掌随手臂缓缓下落，沉肩垂肘，两掌相叠落至脐部丹田部位，同时两膝微屈，缓缓下坐成高位桩。

Exhalation: Slowly drop the arms, relax the shoulders, and drop the elbows. Place the overlapped palms over the Dantian area and slightly flex the knees to make a high-position *Zhan Zhuang*.

图 1-2　Fig 1-2

一呼一吸为1次，共练6~12次。

One respiratory cycle consists of one inhalation and one exhalation and repeat 6–12 cycles.

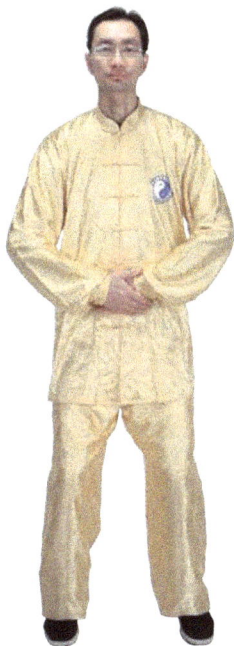

收功：两手相叠抱于丹田，同时屈膝成站桩势，静养丹田半分钟。

Closing posture: Place overlapped hands over the Dantian area, flex the knees to make a *Zhan Zhuang* position and remain still for 30 seconds.

图 1-3　Fig 1-3

第二势　左右托天

Movement # 2　Lift the heaven with both hands

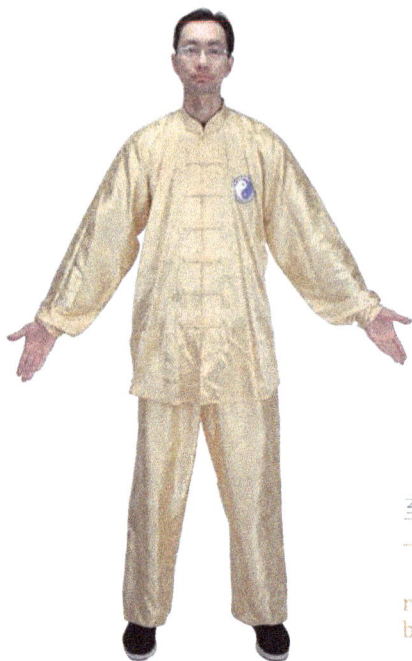

接上势，两掌缓缓松开，下落至两侧胯部。

Further to movement # 1, slowly release the palms and drop to the hip bones on both sides.

图 2-1　Fig 2-1

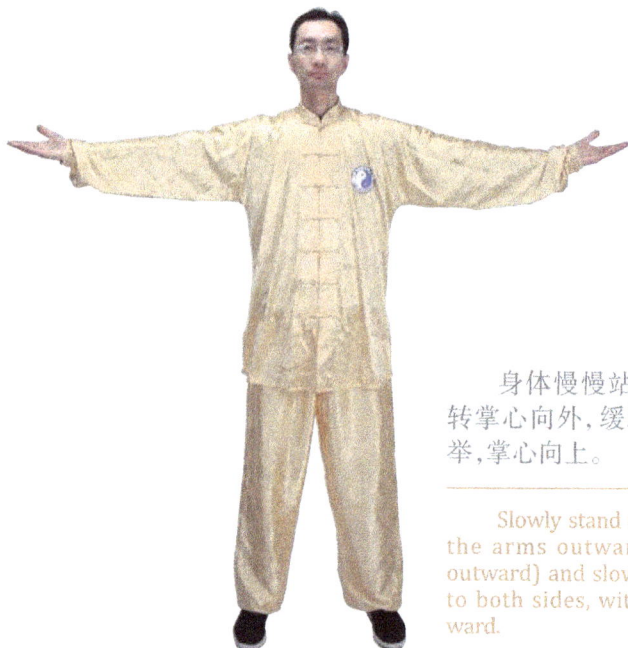

身体慢慢站直，两臂外旋转掌心向外，缓缓上托至侧平举，掌心向上。

Slowly stand up straight. Turn the arms outward (palms also outward) and slowly lift the arms to both sides, with the palms upward.

图 2-2　Fig 2-2

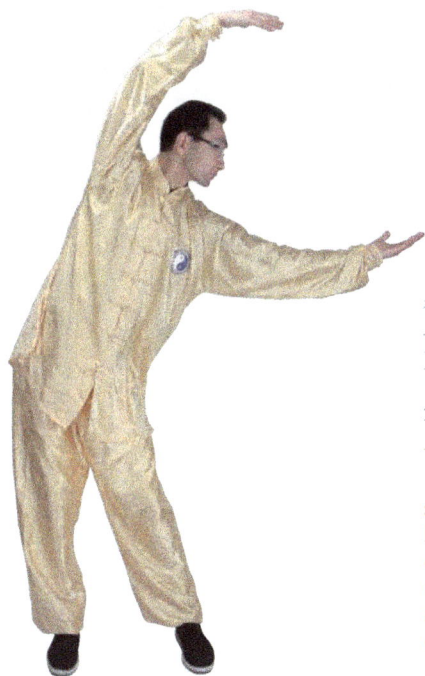

重心略向右移，身体向左侧弯腰，左臂略伸直，右臂上抬至头顶上方略屈，右手心斜对左掌心，两手如抱一气球，眼睛看着左手掌心。

Shift the body weight to the right side, bend to the left side and extend the left arm. Lift the right arm above the top of the head (slightly flexed), make the right palm obliquely facing the left palm as if holding a balloon and focus the eyes on the left palm.

图 2-3　Fig 2-3

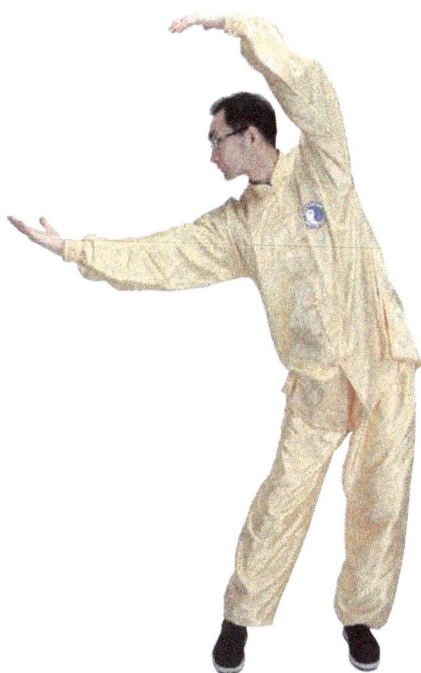

两臂向上抬起，腰部缓缓伸直，再向右侧弯腰，两手掌如捧气球送向右侧，右臂略与肩平，左臂屈于头顶上方，左掌心斜对右手心，眼观右掌心。

Lift the arms, slowly straighten up the low back, and bend to the right side, as if holding a balloon to the right side. Lift the right arm to the level of the shoulder, place the left arm above the top of the head, make the left palm obliquely facing the right palm and focus the eyes on the right palm.

图 2-4　Fig 2-4

一左一右为1次，共练6~12次。

One cycle consists of left side and right side and repeat 6-12 cycles.

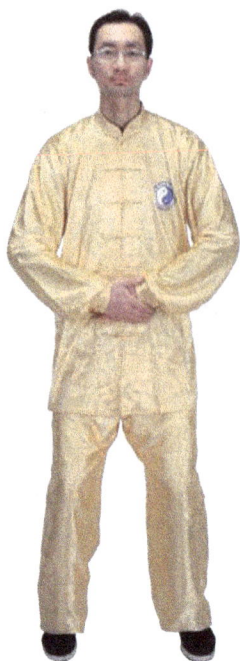

收功：最后一次右侧弯，身体慢慢站直，左臂向左打开，两臂内旋转掌心向前，向前划圆，两掌相叠抱于脐部丹田，同时屈膝成站桩势，静养丹田半分钟。

Closing posture: After bending to the right side, slowly stand up straight, open the left arm to the left, turn the arms inward and palms forward, and draw a circle forward. Place the overlapped palms over the Dantian area, flex the knees to make a *Zhan Zhuang* posture and remain still for 30 seconds.

图 2-5　Fig 2-5

第三势　开胸舒气
Movement # 3　Open up the chest and soothe qi

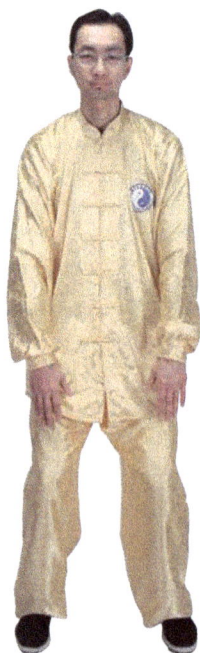

接上势，两掌松开。

Further to movement # 2, release the palms.

图 3-1　Fig 3-1

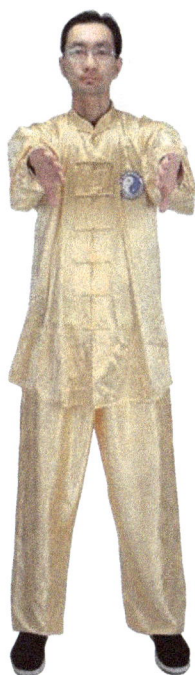

两臂由前上提，同时身体慢慢站直，提至与肩平，同时转掌心向外，手背相对。

Lift the arms from the front of the body and slowly stand up straight. Turn the palms outward when the arms are at the level of the shoulders and make the dorsa of the hands facing each other.

图 3-2　Fig 3-2

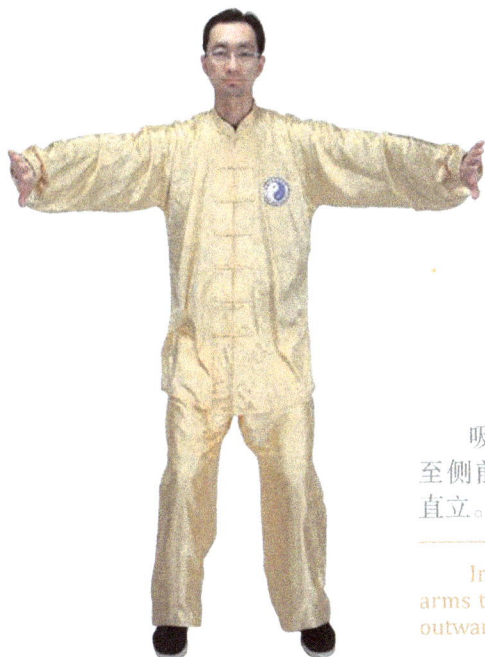

吸气，两臂慢慢向左右分开至侧前方，掌心向外，保持身体直立。

Inhalation: Slowly separate the arms to both sides, make the palms outward, and keep the body upright.

图 3-3　Fig 3-3

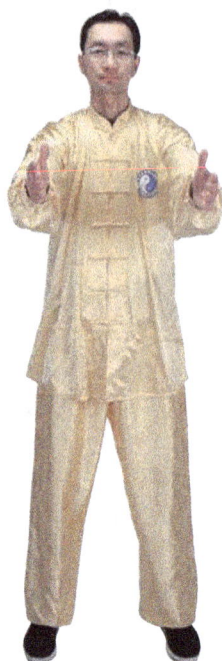

呼气，两臂外旋转掌心向内，缓缓向内合拢至胸前，掌心相对略与肩宽，同时屈膝下坐成站桩。

Exhalation: Turn the arms outward (palms inward), slowly fold the arms in front of the chest, make the palms facing each other at shoulder-width apart and flex the knees into a *Zhan Zhuang* posture.

图 3-4　Fig 3-4

一呼一吸为1次，共练6~12次。

One respiratory cycle consists of one inhalation and one exhalation and repeat 6–12 cycles.

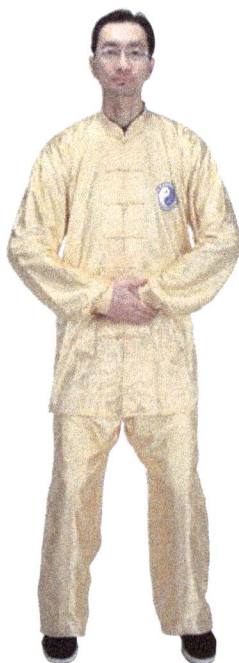

收功：最后一次结束，屈肘转掌心向内，两掌相叠抱于脐部丹田，同时屈膝成站桩势，静养丹田半分钟。

Closing posture: Flex the elbows, turn the palms inward, place the overlapped palms over the Dantian area, flex the knees into a *Zhan Zhuang* posture and remain still for 30 seconds.

图 3-5　Fig 3-5

第四势　丹田划圆
Movement # 4　Draw circles around the Dantian

前划圆
Forward circle

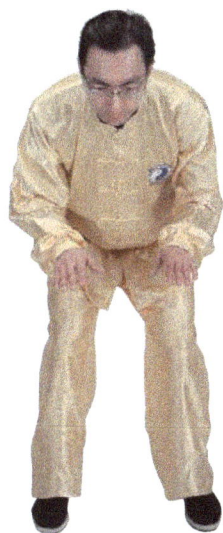

图 4-1　Fig 4-1

接上势，两手慢慢分开向前伸出。

Further to movement # 3, slowly separate the hands and extend forward (palms downward).

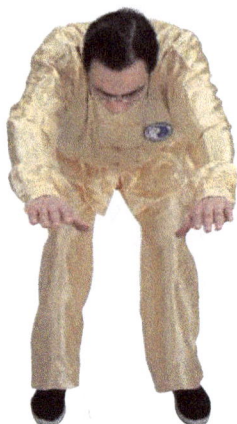

正面　Front view

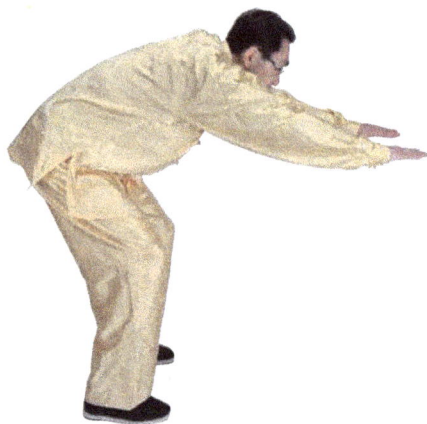

侧面　Side view

图 4-2　Fig 4-2

掌心向下,同时略下坐,上身前倾,至身体前方两掌慢慢向两侧划圆。

Slightly flex the knees and bend the upper body forward, draw circles from front of the body to both sides using the palms until the hip bones.

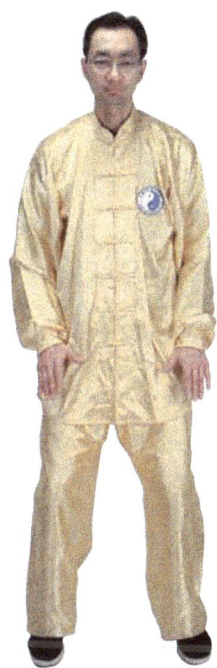

正面　Front view　　　側面　Side view

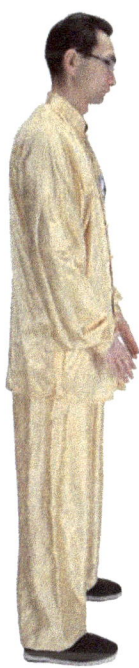

图 4–3　Fig 4–3

收至两侧胯部前，同时身体慢慢站起。

Then slowly stand up.

共练6次划圆。

Forward circles repeat 6 times.

后划圆
Backward circle

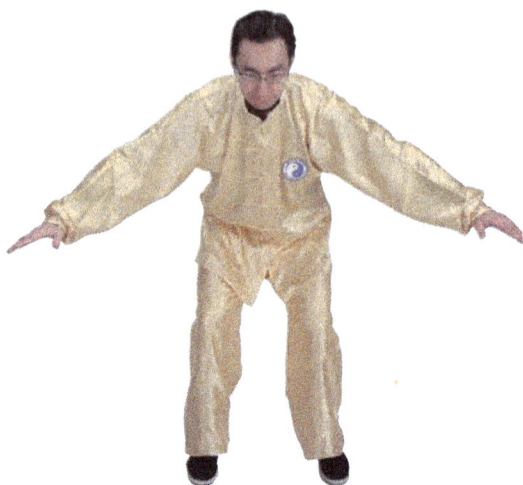

正面　Front view

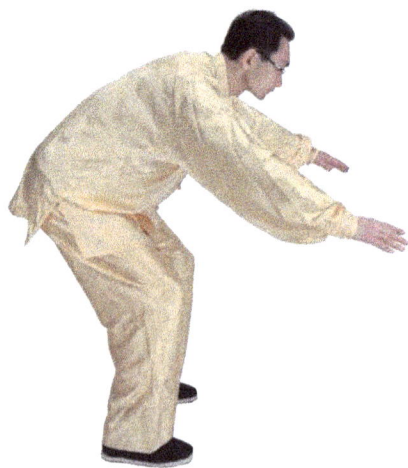

侧面　Side view

图 4-4　Fig 4-4

　　两手由胯前向后划圆、由两侧向前划，掌心向下，同时下坐上身略前倾。

　　From front of the hip bones, draw circles backward, make the palms downward, flex the knees and slightly bend the upper body forward.

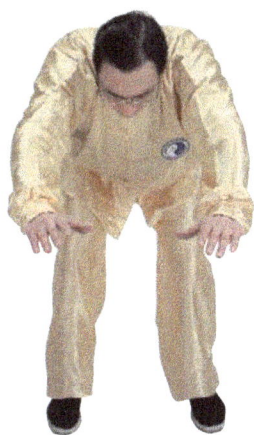

再由前回收至两胯前。

Return the hands to the hip bones.

图 4-5　Fig 4-5

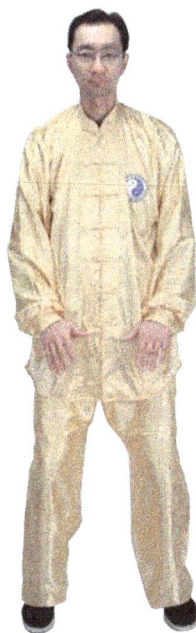

同时身体慢慢站起。

Slowly stand up.

图 4-6　Fig 4-6

共练6次划圆。

Backward circle repeat 6 times.

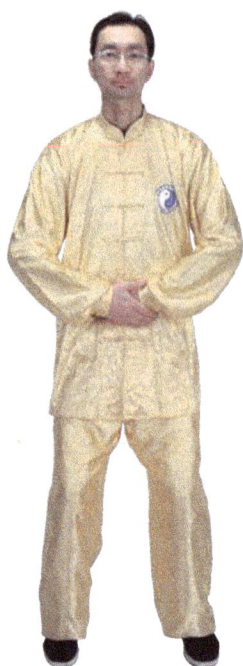

收功：最后一次后划圆结束，身体慢慢站起，转掌心向内对准丹田，两掌相叠抱于脐部丹田，同时屈膝成站桩势，静养丹田半分钟。

Closing posture: After drawing the last circle, slowly stand up, turn the palms inward to face Dantian, place the overlapped palms over the Dantian area, flex the knees into a *Zhan Zhuang* posture and remain still for 30 seconds.

图 4-7　Fig 4-7

第五势　双手按膝
Movement # 5　Press the knees with both hands

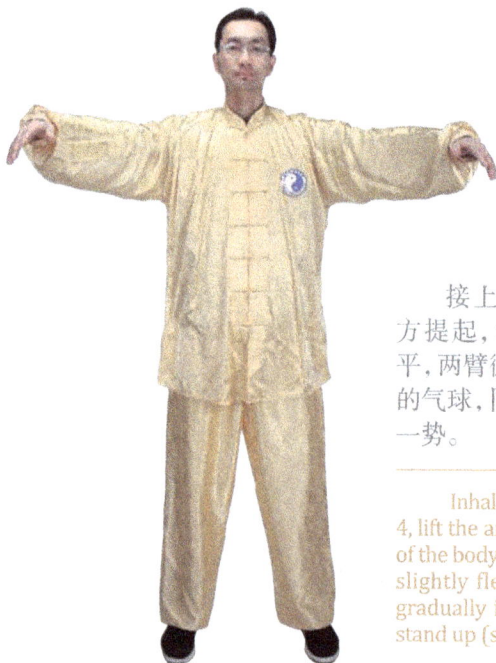

接上势。吸气，两臂由侧前方提起，掌心向下，至手掌与肩平，两臂微曲，如抱一个缓缓涨大的气球，同时身体慢慢站直，同第一势。

Inhalation: Further to movement # 4, lift the arms from anterolateral sides of the body, make the palms downward, slightly flex the arms as if holding a gradually inflated balloon and slowly stand up (same as movement # 1).

图 5-1　Fig 5-1

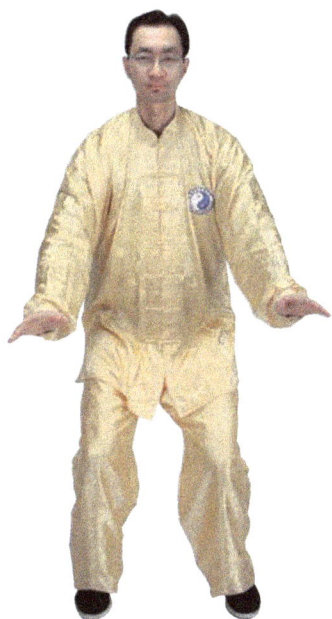

呼气，身体慢慢下坐，两臂下落。

Exhalation: Slowly flex the knees, drop the arms.

图 5-2　Fig 5-2

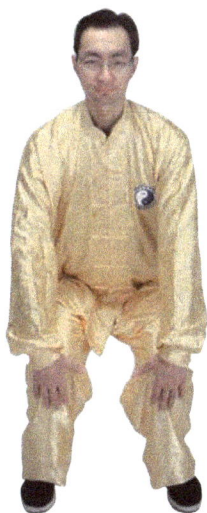

两掌轻轻按于两膝关节上。

Gently press the knee joints with the palms.

图 5-3　Fig 5-3

一呼一吸为1次，共练6~12次。

One respiratory cycle consists of one inhalation and one exhalation and repeat 6–12 cycles.

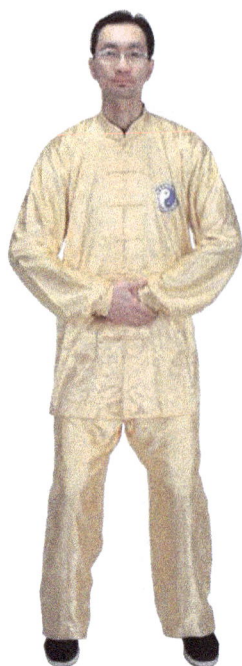

收功：最后一次按膝结束，身体慢慢站起，两臂上提，转掌心向内对准丹田，两掌相叠抱于脐部丹田，同时屈膝成站桩势，静养丹田半分钟。

Closing posture: After the last time of pressing the knee joints, slowly stand up, lift the arms, turn the palms inward to face Dantian, place the overlapped palms over the Dantian area, flex the knees into a *Zhan Zhuang* posture and remain still for 30 seconds.

图 5-4　Fig 5-4

第六势　升降开合
Movement # 6　Ascend, descend, open and close

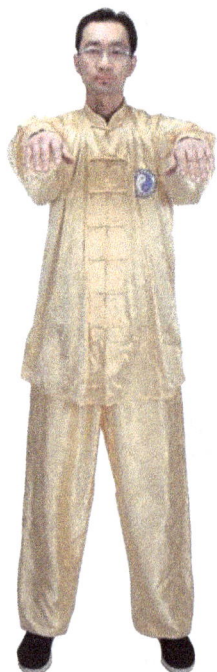

接上势。吸气，两臂由前慢慢上提至与肩平、手心向下，保持臂腕放松，身体渐渐站直。

Inhalation: Further to movement # 5, slowly lift the arms from the front of the body to the level of the shoulders, make the palms downward, relax the arms and wrists and slowly stand up straight.

图 6-1　Fig 6-1

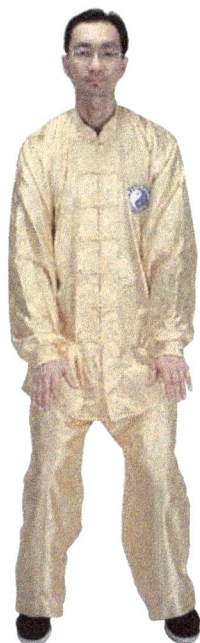

呼气，身体慢慢下坐，同时沉
肩垂肘屈臂下落至大腿前。

Exhalation: Slowly flex the
knees, relax the shoulders, drop the
elbows and flex the arms to the front
of the thigh.

图 6-2　Fig 6-2

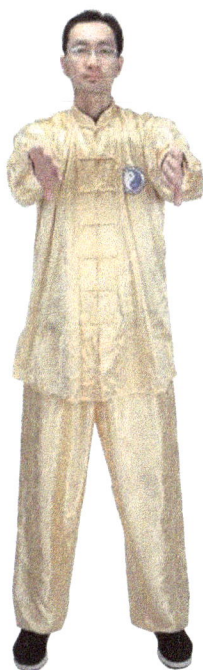

吸气，两臂由前上提同时转
掌心向外，手背相对，缓缓向外
分开。

Inhalation: Lift the arms from
the front of the body, turn the palms
outward, make the dorsa of the hands
facing each other. Slowly separate
them outward.

图 6-3　Fig 6-3

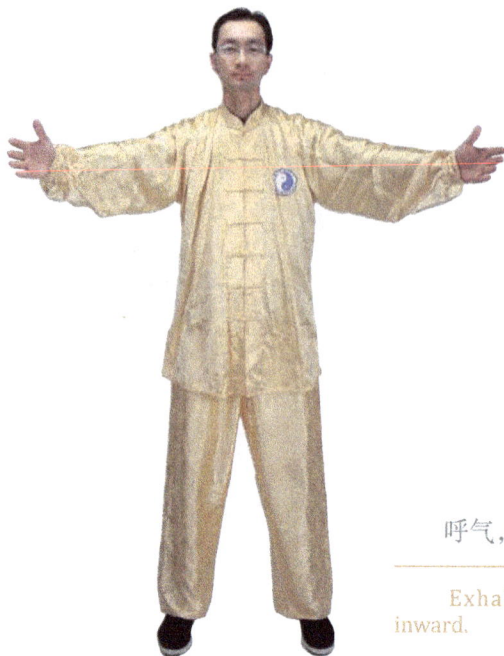

呼气,转掌心向内。

Exhalation: Turn the palms inward.

图 6-4   Fig 6-4

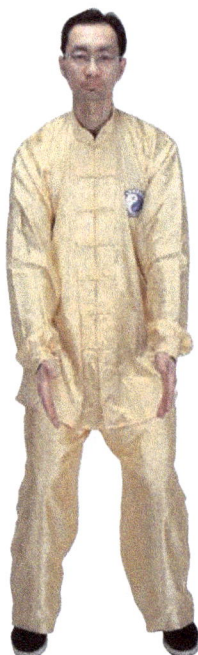

两臂内合,合至胸前慢慢下落,落至大腿前,手心相对。

Put the arms together and slowly drop the arms from the front of the chest to the front of the thigh, making the palms facing each other.

图 6-5   Fig 6-5

二吸二呼为1次,共练3~6次。

One respiratory cycle consists of one inhalation and one exhalation and repeat 3–6 cycles.

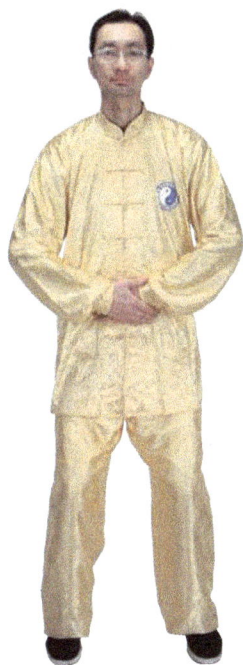

收功：最后一次练习结束，身体慢慢站起，两臂外旋，由两侧缓缓向前合拢，两掌相叠抱于脐部丹田，同时屈膝成站桩势，静养丹田半分钟。

Closing posture: After the last exercise, slowly stand up, turn the arms outward and put the arms together from both sides to the front of the body. Place the overlapped palms over the Dantian area, flex the knees into a *Zhan Zhuang* posture and remain still for 30 seconds.

图 6-6　Fig 6-6

收势
Concluding posture

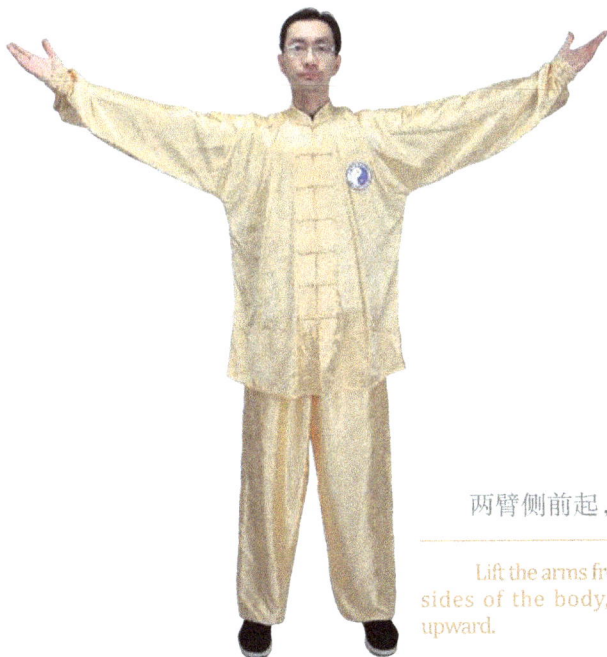

两臂侧前起，掌心向上。

Lift the arms from the anterolateral sides of the body, make the palms upward.

收势图1　Concluding posture 1

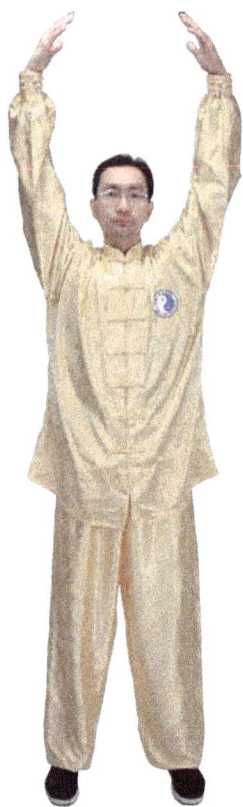

缓缓升至头顶、气贯百汇。

Slowly lift the palms above the top of the head to send qi to Baihui (DU 20) point.

收势图2　Concluding posture 2

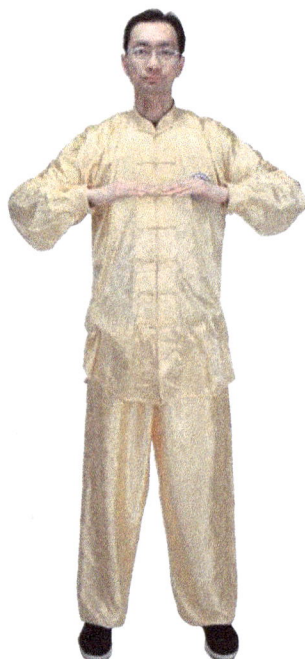

两臂屈肘，掌心下按，由体前慢慢下按至小腹。

Flex the elbows, press the palms down from front of the body to the lower abdomen.

收势图3　Concluding posture 3

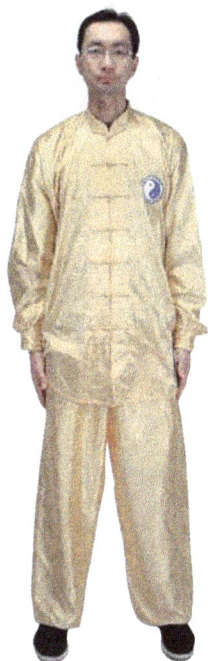

分手还原，收左脚成并步站立。

Separate the hands, retract the left foot and stand with the feet together.

收势图4　Concluding posture 4

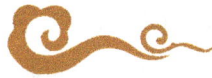

逍 遥 功　　•　　*Xiao Yao Gong* (Free and Easy Exercise)

Application

应用

现代实验研究证明，在练功放松入静时，可见到练功者脑电图中α波波幅增高，并由枕叶逐渐向颞叶扩散；单位时间氧耗明显下降。由于α波是反映大脑皮层抑制的波型，所以α波波幅增高，并有扩散趋势。说明气功锻炼可减轻或消除大脑皮层各种不良刺激，可调节中枢神经，促进大脑皮层和全身脏器得到休养生息，提高记忆能力或开发智力。长期气功锻炼，又能够双向调节各系统功能，还能促进血液循环，增强心脏的功能，对防治冠心病、脑动脉硬化等心脑血管病和其他血液循环障碍的病症都有良好作用。

Laboratory studies have shown that, during qigong practice, the brain α wave amplitude in EEG was elevated and gradually spread from the occipital lobe toward the temporal lobe, coupled with a significant drop in oxygen consumption. Since α waves reflect the inhibition of cerebral cortex, their elevated amplitude and tendency to spread suggest that qigong can alleviate or eliminate pessimal stimulation to cerebral cortex, regulate central nervous system, recuperate the cerebral cortex and internal organs and improve memory and intelligence. Over time, qigong practice can regulate functions of the body systems, increase blood circulation, benefit the heart and thus prevent or treat cardio-cerebrovascular diseases (such as coronary artery disease and cerebral arteriosclerosis) and disturbance of blood circulation.

疏 通 经 络

Unblocks meridians

经络是气血运行的通路。经络不通则痛，脏腑组织器官得不到气血的滋养和温煦，导致各种病症。通过本功法的习练可有效促进经络疏通，具体如左右托天势可疏通两侧胆经和督脉；开胸舒气势能疏通肺经与心脉等；丹田划圆势可以开通代脉，调理下焦；升降开合势可以开通任脉与冲脉等。经络通则不痛，脏腑组织就能得到气血的供应，减轻或消除各种慢性病症。

Meridians are pathways of qi and blood circulation. Other than pain, obstruction of meridians results in failure of qi and blood to nourish and warm zang-fu organs and tissues. Practice of *Xiao Yao Gong* can effectively unblock meridians. For example, movement # 2 (Lift the heaven with both hands) unblocks the gallbladder and *Du* meridians, movement # 3 (Open up the chest and soothe qi) unblocks the lung and heart meridians, movement # 4 (Draw circles around the Dantian) unblocks *Dai*[1] meridians and regulate the lower *jiao* and movement # 6 (Ascend, descend, open and close) unblocks *Ren* and *Chong* meridians. Other than pain relief, unblocked meridians can guarantee supply of qi and blood to zang-fu organs and tissues and thus alleviate or eliminate chronic problems.

调 和 气 血

Harmonizes qi and blood

气血是滋养人体的营养物质。如果气血不足就可导致贫血或营养不良，免疫功能下降，就产生许多虚证病候；如果气滞血瘀就可导致气血运行障碍，会产生许多实证病候。通过习练本功法，不仅可以补益气血，而且又可理气活血，所以能够防治虚证和实证的许多病症。

Since qi and blood nurtures our body, insufficient qi and

---

1. One of the eight extraordinary meridians that goes round the waist like a belt binding the yin and yang meridians.

blood may result in anemia/malnutrition, weakened immune system and deficiency symptoms; qi stagnation and blood stasis may disturb circulation of qi and blood and result in excess symptoms. Practice of *Xiao Yao Gong* can not only supplement qi and nourish blood, but also regulate qi and circulate blood, thus improving both deficiency and excess symptoms.

形 神 合 一
Integrates body with mind

　　本功法动中寓静，秉承道家逍遥游的精神，充分体现了道家清净、自然、无为、柔弱的特点，通过形体的外在导引，配合呼吸、意识的运用，让形神逐渐相融相合，并进而忘却身心，使身心进入一种逍遥自在的玄妙的气功状态，如长期习练可以提升生命的质量与境界。

By integrating active body movements with inner cultivation, *Xiao Yao Gong* contains the Daoist spirit of free and easy wandering and presents Daoist characteristics of pureness, at ease, inaction and softness. Through combination of physical *Dao Yin* with breathing and mental consciousness, practice of *Xiao Yao Gong* can gradually help you to enter an amazing qigong state, which unites your body and mind and free yourself from the world. In the long term, this exercise can improve the quality and realm of your life.

防 病 治 病
Prevents and treats disease

　　通过长期的教学与临床实践证明，本功法锻炼既可扶助正气，又可祛除邪气，并且能起到舒肝解郁、舒缓身心的作用，所以能够防治如冠心病、心律不齐、老慢支、多种心理疾病以及胃病等多种慢性疾病。具体为：习练吐纳炼丹势可以增强丹田内气，防治肠胃道等消化系统疾病；左右托天势可防治冠心病、老慢支、心律不齐等心肺系统疾病；开胸舒气势可防治冠心病、高血压、心律不齐等心血管疾病；丹田划圆势可防治泌尿生殖系统疾病如慢性肾炎、膀胱炎等。另外双手按膝势可防治身体虚弱、腿脚无力；而升降开合势可通调全身脏腑的气机，使身心更和谐。

Teaching and clinical practice have proven that *Xiao Yao Gong* can reinforce healthy qi, remove pathogenic factors, soothe liver qi and relax the body and mind. Long-term practice of *Xiao Yao Gong* can prevent and treat mental problems and chronic conditions including coronary artery disease, cardiac arrhythmias, chronic bronchitis, and stomach diseases. Specifically, movement # 1 (Strengthen Dantian through breathing) strengthens internal qi in Dantian and prevents gastrointestinal disorders; movement # 2 (Lift the heaven with both hands) prevents cardiopulmonary problems such as coronary artery disease, chronic bronchitis and cardiac arrhythmias; movement # 3 (Open up the chest and soothe qi) prevents cardiovascular diseases such as coronary artery disease, hypertension and cardiac arrhythmias; and movement # 4 (Draw circles around the Dantian) prevents urogenital problems such as chronic nephritis and cystitis. In addition, movement # 5 (Press the knees with both hands) prevents weakness of the body and legs, and movement 6 (Ascend, descend, open and close) regulates qi activities of the zang-fu organs and harmonize the body and mind.

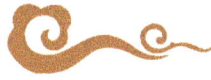

逍 遥 功 ● *Xiao Yao Gong* (Free and Easy Exercise)

The Meridian Charts

经络图

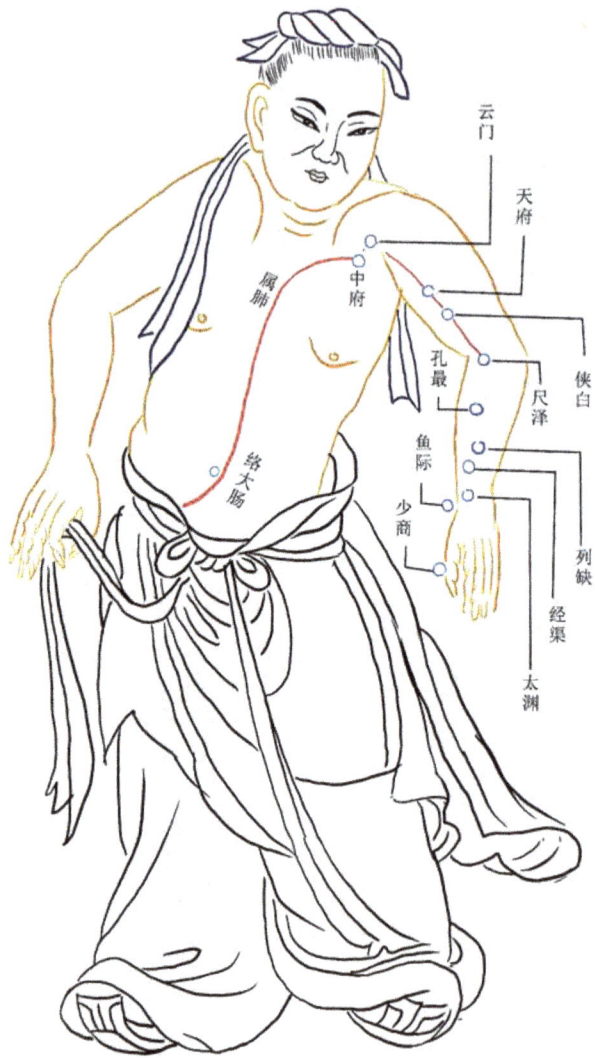

云门
天府
侠白
列缺
经渠
太渊
中府
属肺
孔最
尺泽
鱼际
少商
络大肠

手太阴肺经

Lung Meridian of Hand-Taiyin

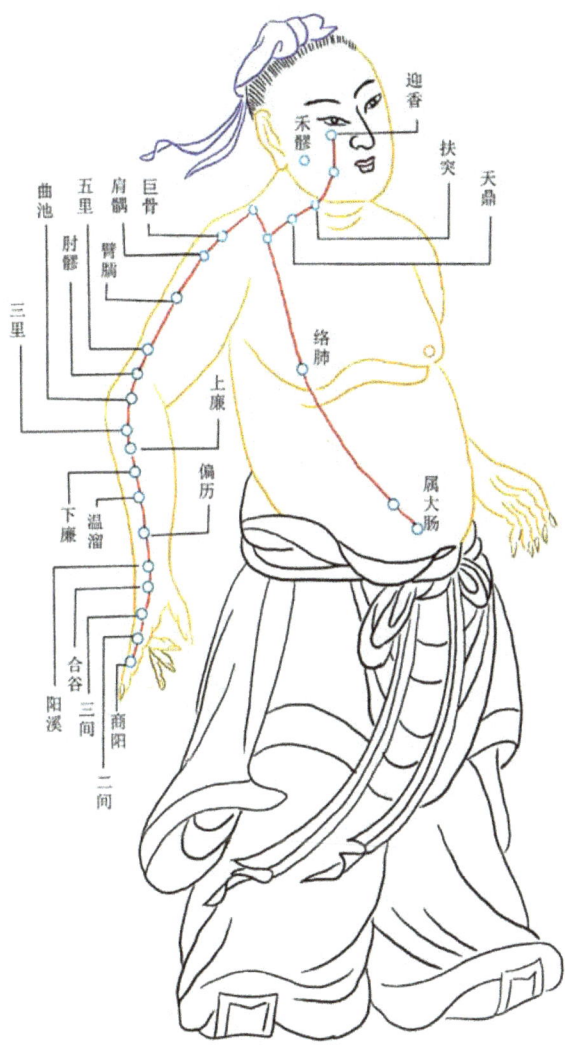

迎香
禾髎
扶突
天鼎
巨骨
肩髃
五里
曲池
臂臑
肘髎
三里
络肺
上廉
偏历
属大肠
下廉
温溜
合谷
阳溪
三间
商阳
二间

手阳明大肠经

Large Intestine Meridian of Hand-Yangming

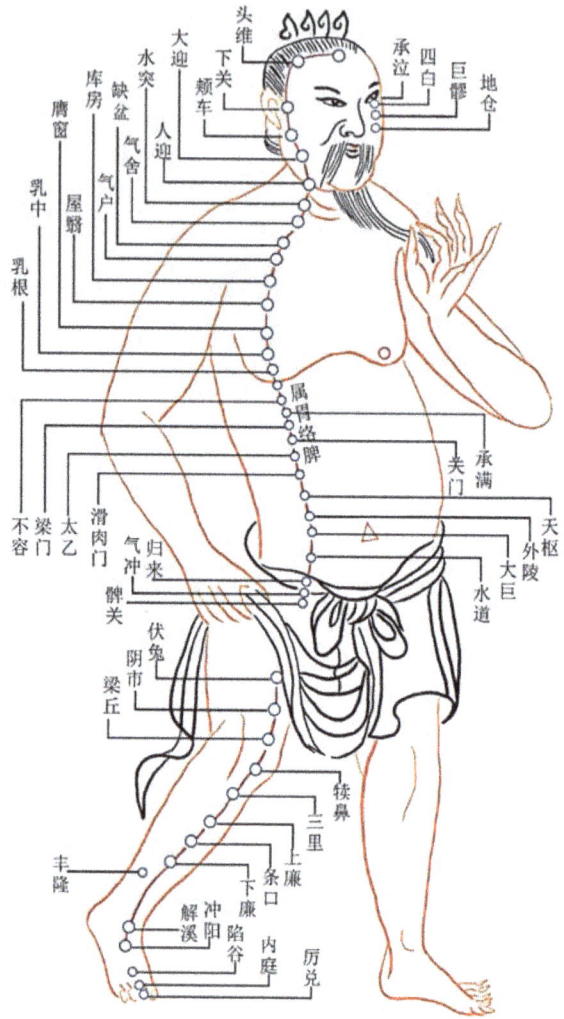

头维 下关 颊车 人迎 水突 大迎 缺盆 气舍 气户 库房 膺窗 屋翳 乳中 乳根 承泣 四白 巨髎 地仓 属胃络脾 承满 关门 天枢 外陵 大巨 水道 归来 气冲 髀关 伏兔 阴市 梁丘 滑肉门 太乙 梁门 不容 犊鼻 三里 上廉 条口 下廉 冲阳 陷谷 内庭 厉兑 丰隆 解溪

足阳明胃经

Stomach Meridian of Foot-Yangming

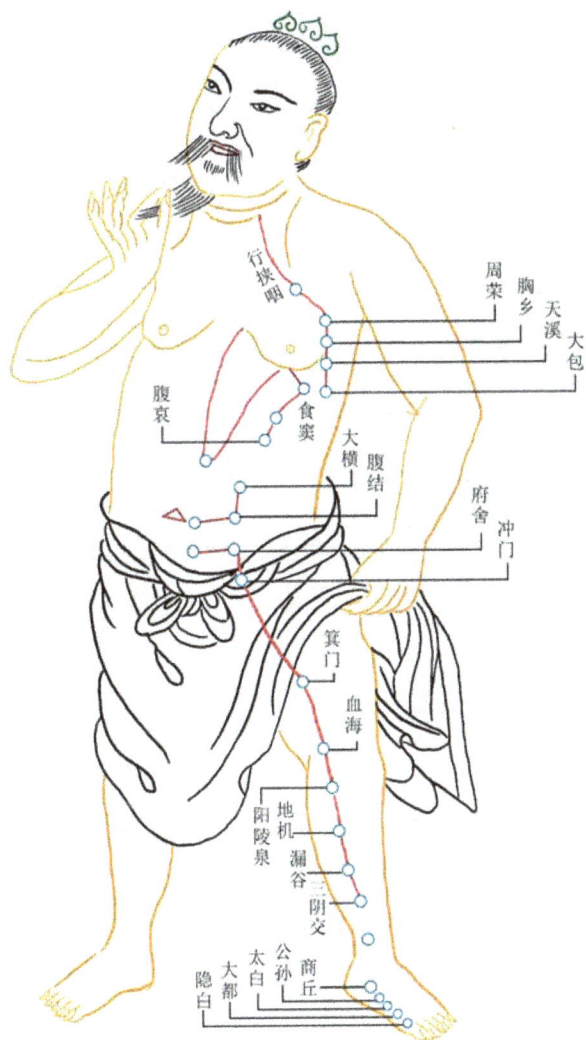

足太阴脾经

Spleen Meridian of Foot-Taiyin

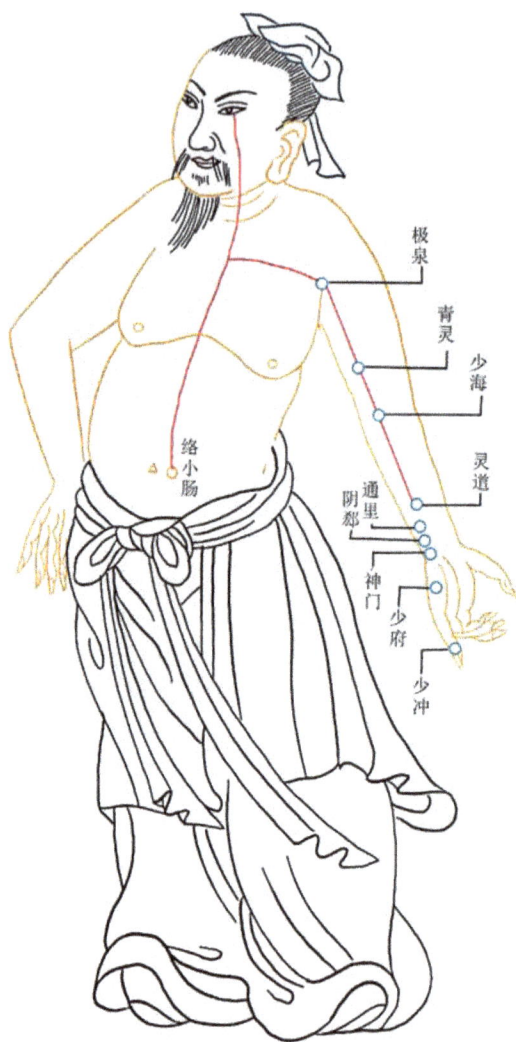

极泉
青灵
少海
灵道
通里
阴郄
神门
少府
少冲
络 小肠

手少阴心经

Heart Meridian of Hand-Shaoyin

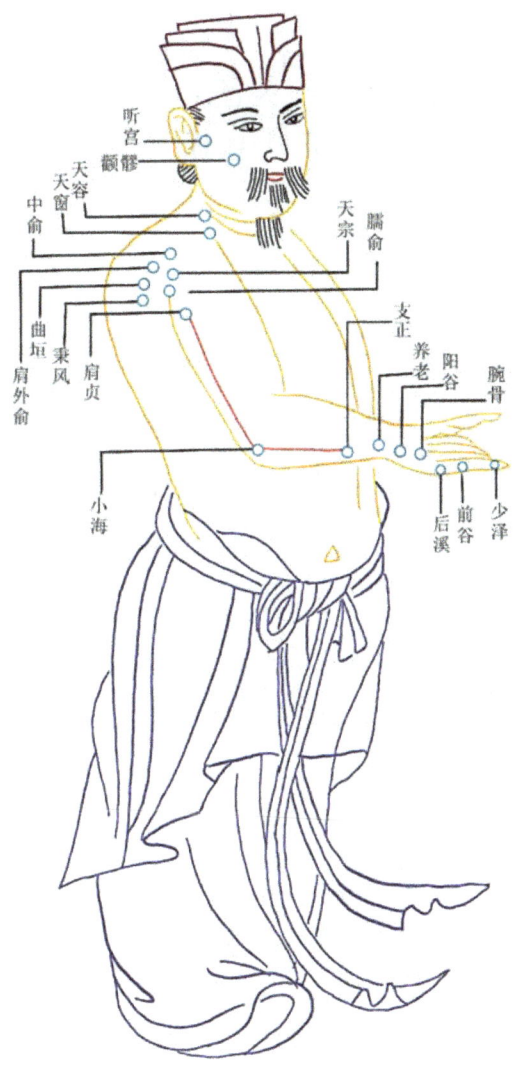

听宫
颧髎
天容
天窗
中俞
曲垣
秉风
肩贞
肩外俞
小海
天宗
膈俞
支正
养老
阳谷
腕骨
少泽
前谷
后溪

手太阳小肠经

Small Intestine Meridian of Hand-Taiyang

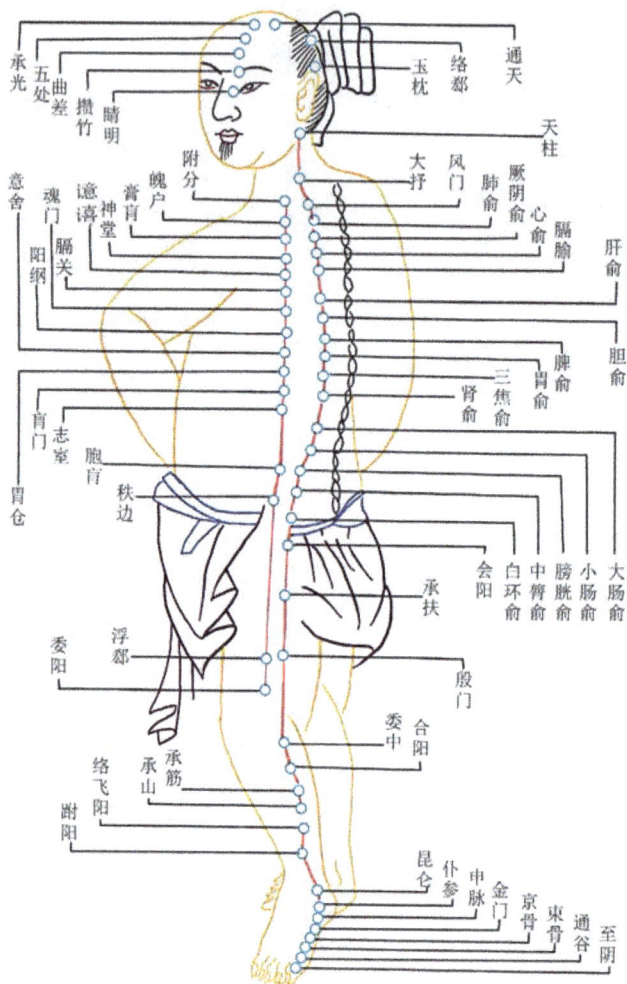

足太阳膀胱经

Bladder Meridian of Foot-Taiyang

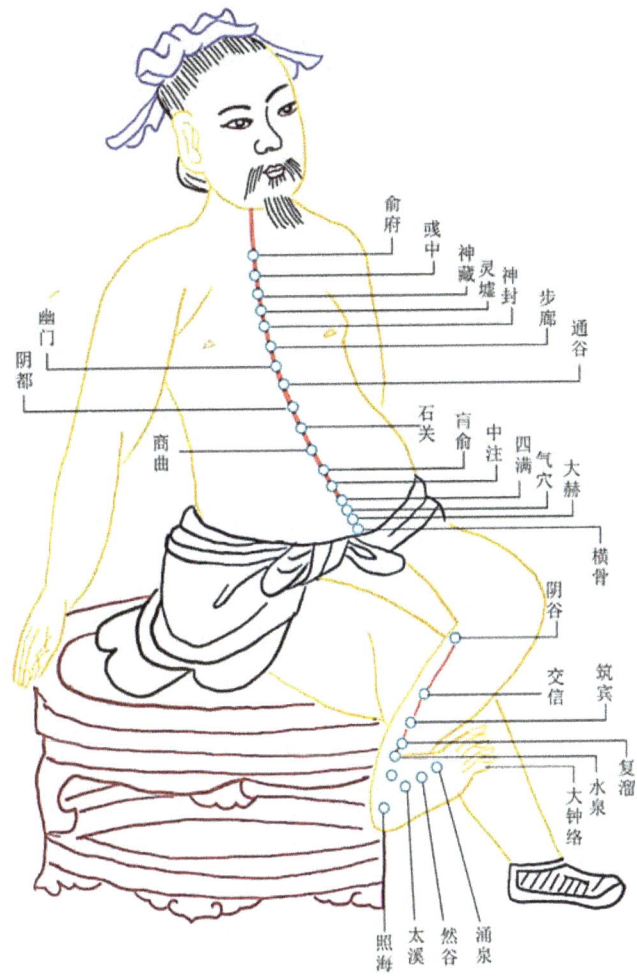

足少阴肾经

Kidney Meridian of Foot-Shaoyin

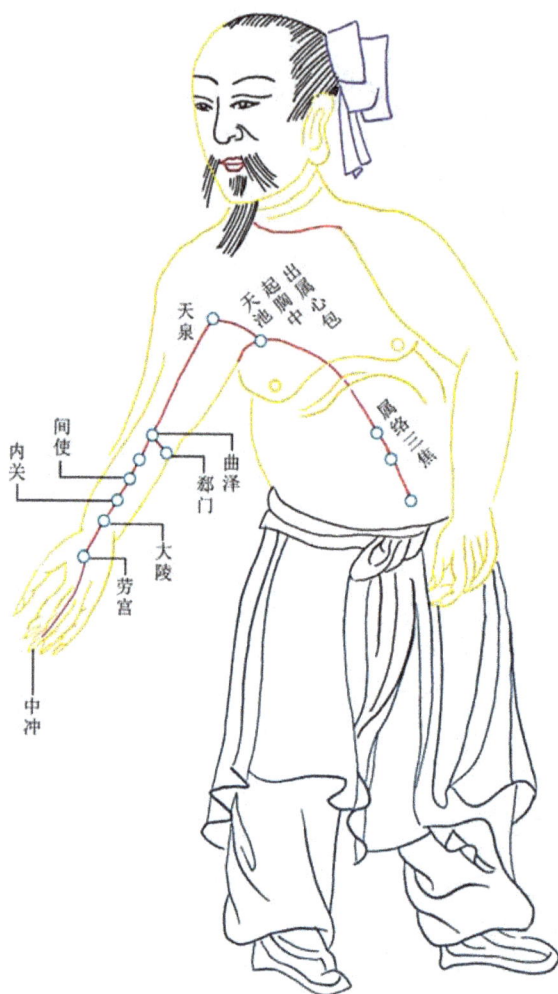

天泉

天起属心包
池出属胸中

间使

内关

曲泽
郄门

大陵

劳宫

属络三焦

中冲

手厥阴心包经

Pericardium Meridian of Hand-Jueyin

手少阳三焦经

Triple Energizer Meridian of Hand-Shaoyang

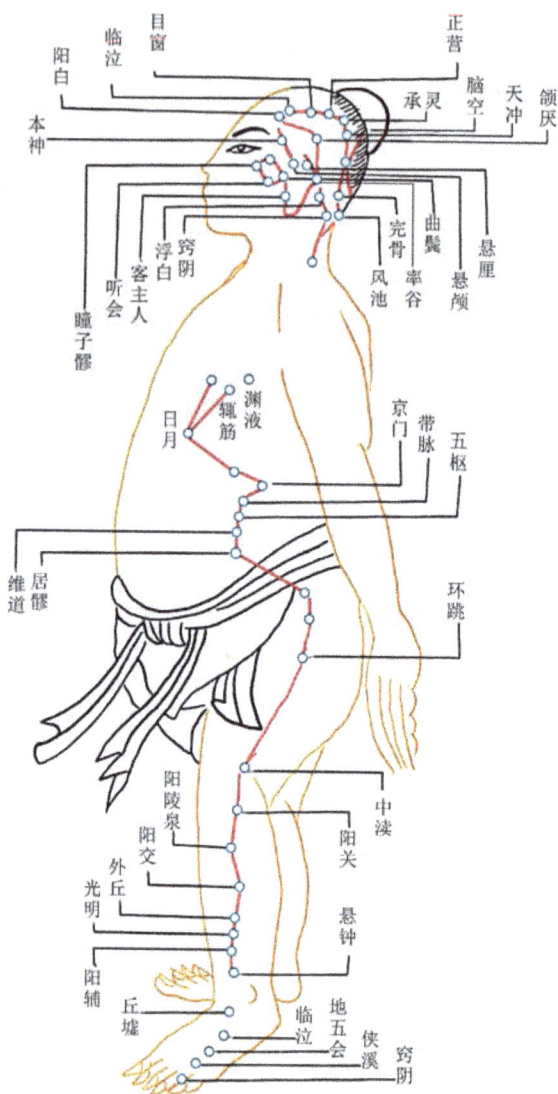

足少阳胆经

Gallbladder Meridian of Foot-Shaoyang

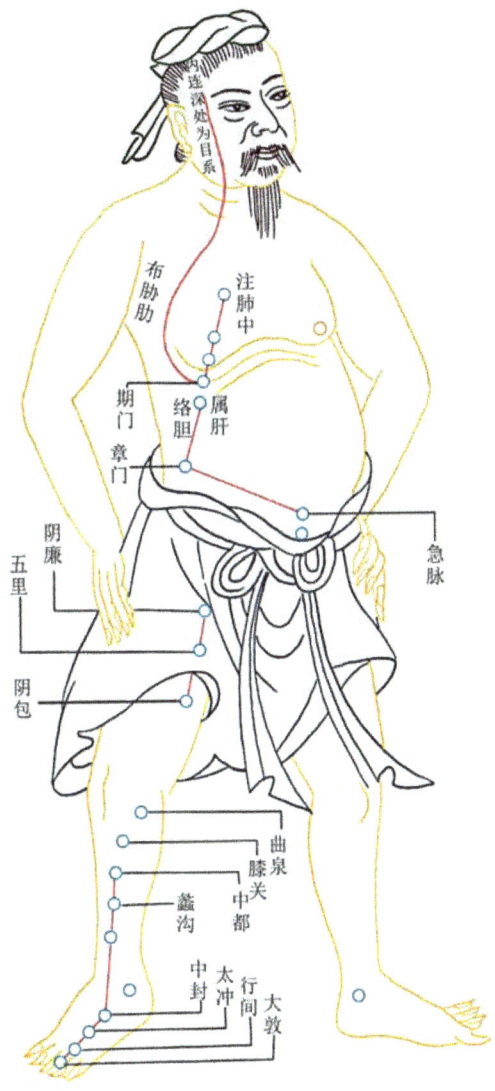

足厥阴肝经

Liver Meridian of Foot-Jueyin

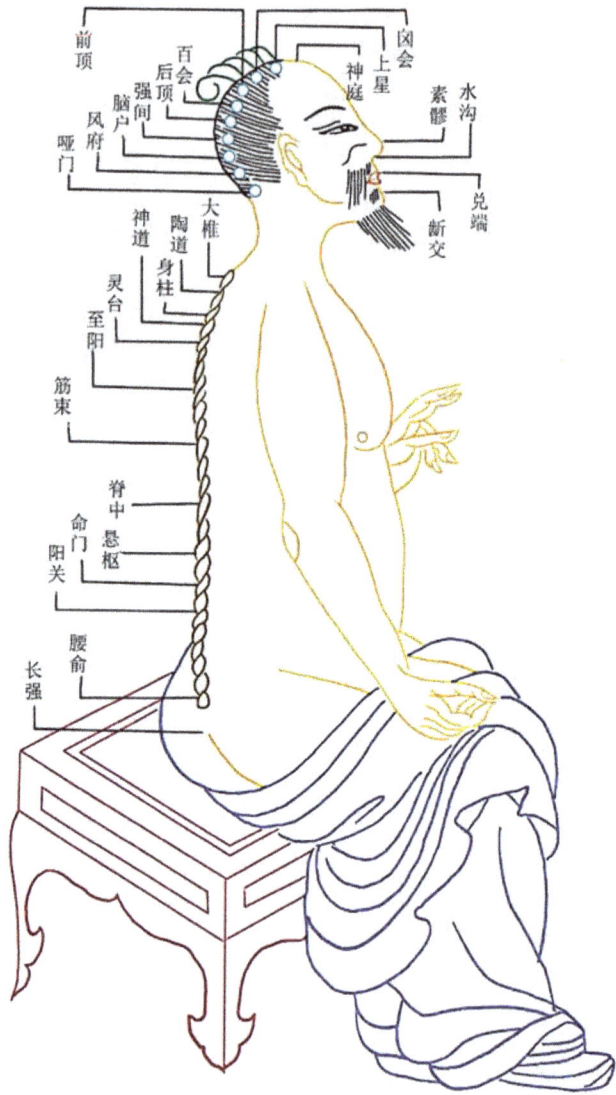

督脉

Governor Vessel (Du)

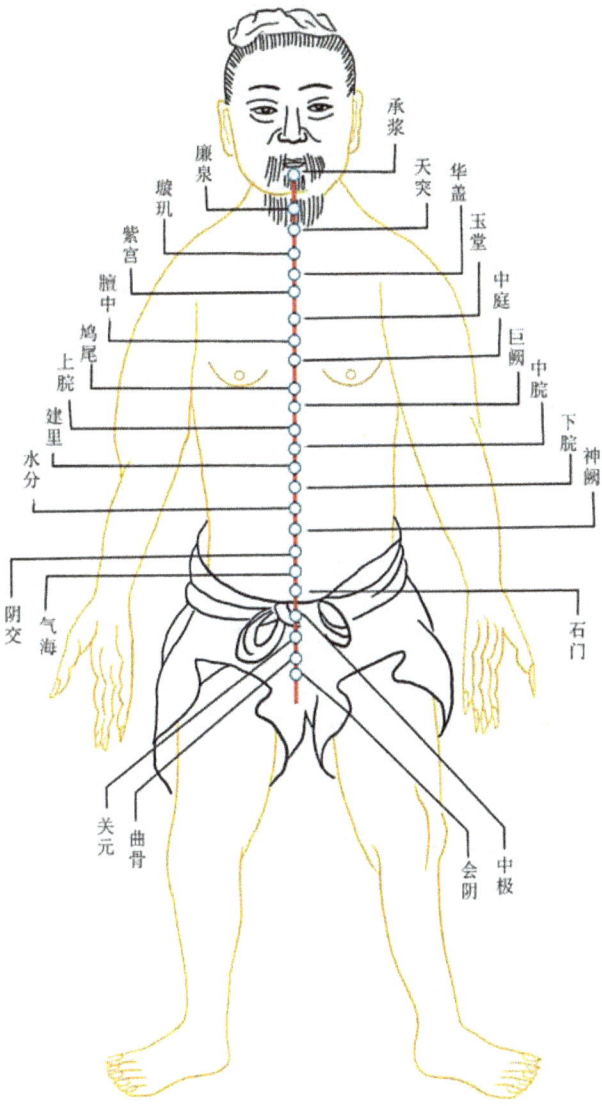

承浆
廉泉
璇玑
紫宫
膻中
鸠尾
上脘
建里
水分
阴交
气海
关元
曲骨
会阴
中极
石门
神阙
下脘
中脘
巨阙
中庭
玉堂
华盖
天突

任脉

Conception Vessel (Ren)

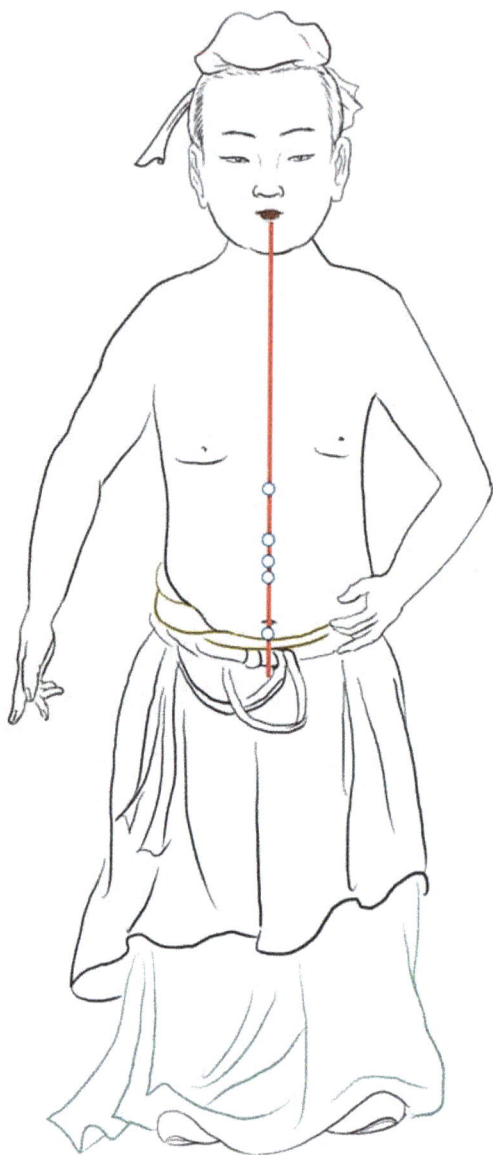

冲脉

Thoroughfare Vessel (Chong)

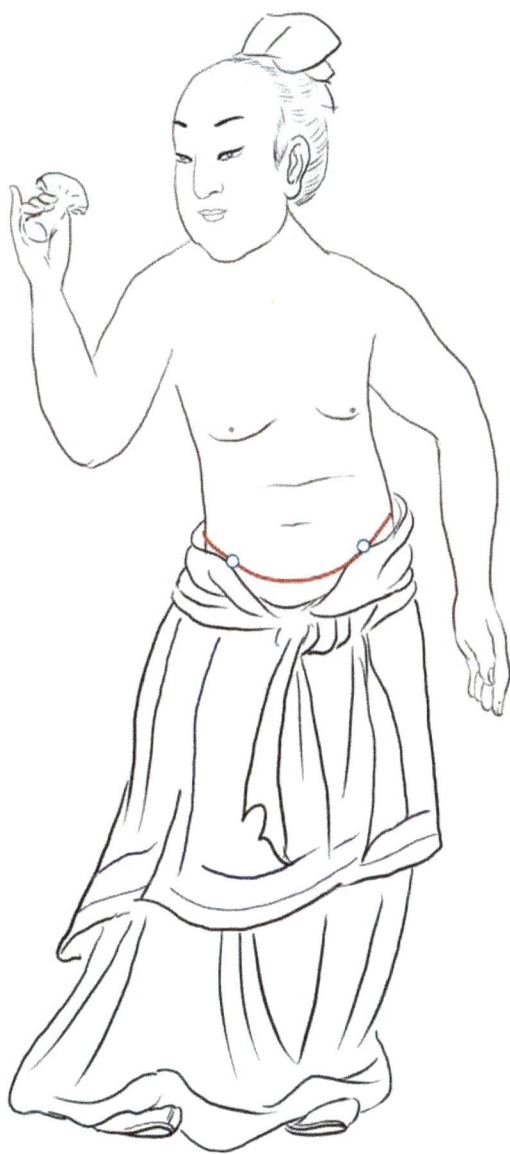

带脉

Belt Vessel (Dai)

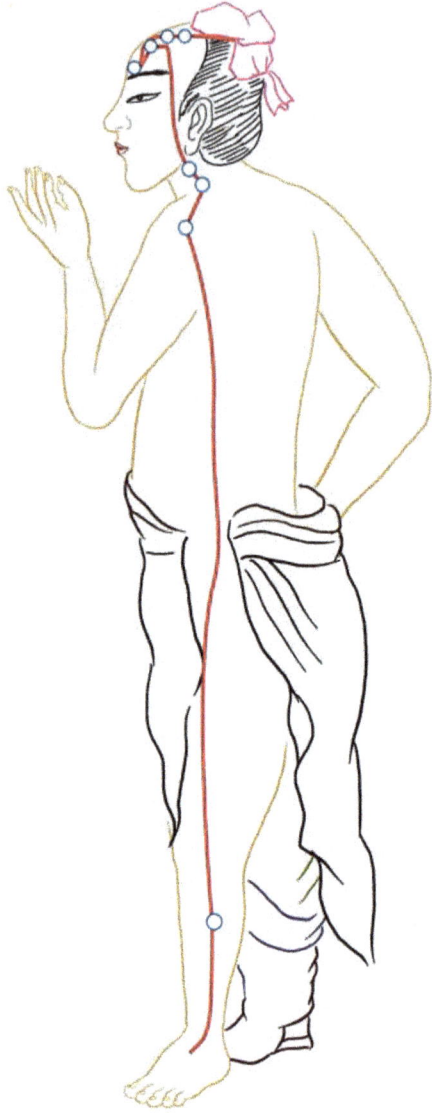

阳维脉

Yang Link Vessel (Yang Wei)

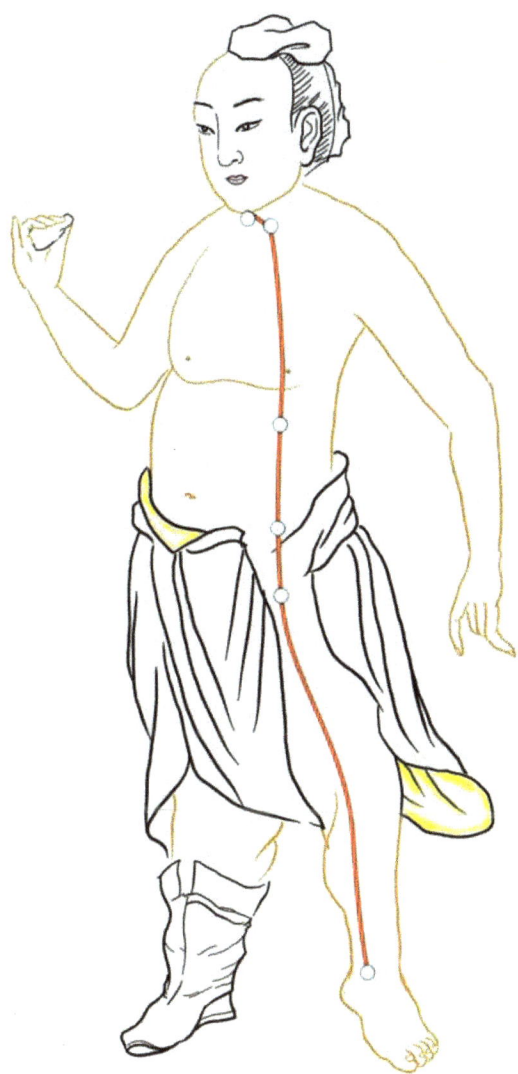

阴维脉

Yin Link Vessel (Yin Wei)

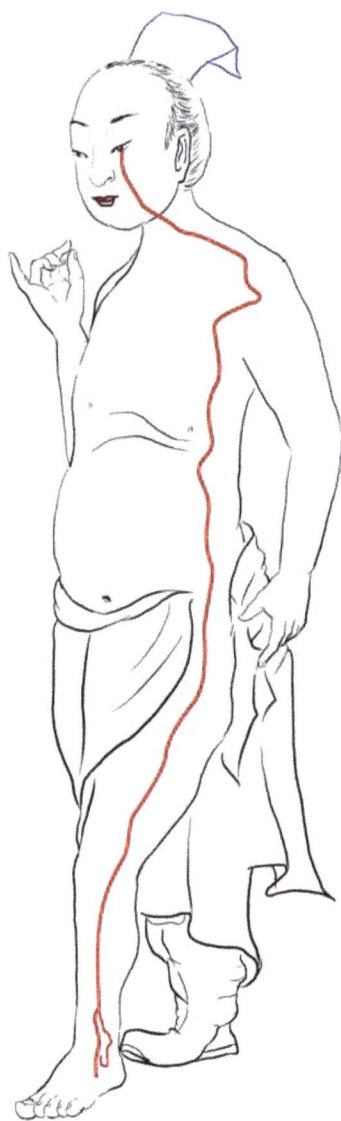

阳蹻脉

Yang Heel Vessel (Yang Qiao)

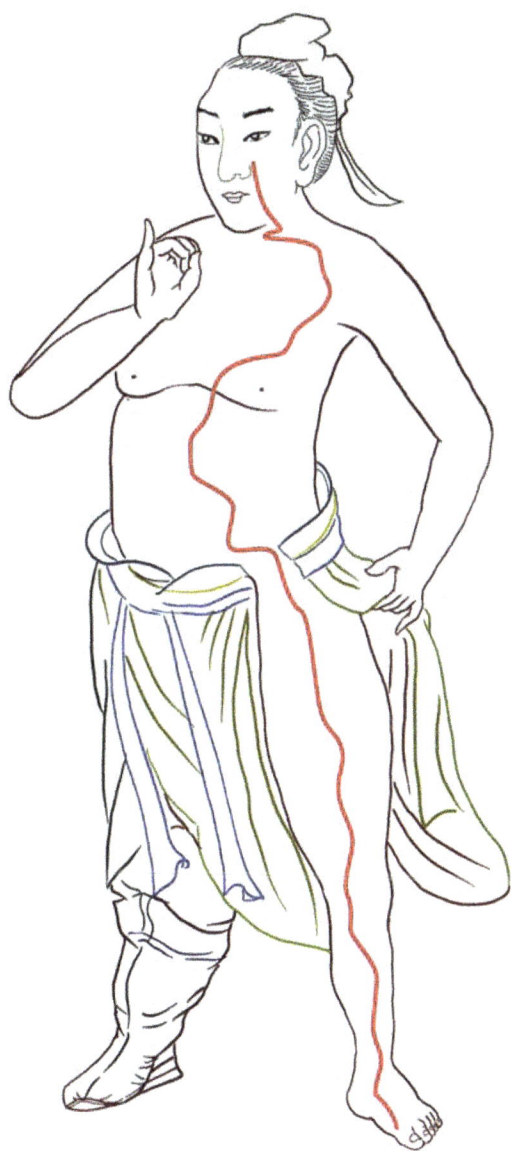

阴跷脉

Yin Heel Vessel (Yin Qiao)

www.ingramcontent.com/pod-product-compliance
Lightning Source LLC
Chambersburg PA
CBHW080053280326
41934CB00014B/3302